About the NCCN Guidelines for Patients®

National Comprehensive Cancer Network®

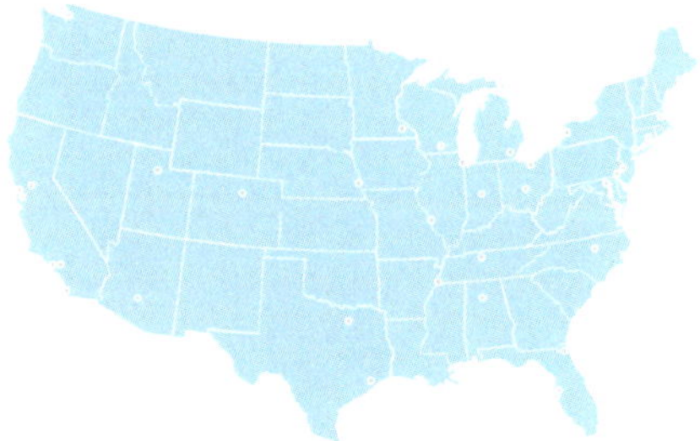

Did you know that top cancer centers across the United States work together to improve cancer care? This alliance of leading cancer centers is called the National Comprehensive Cancer Network® (NCCN®).

Cancer care is always changing. NCCN develops evidence-based cancer care recommendations used by health care providers worldwide. These frequently updated recommendations are the NCCN Clinical Practice Guidelines in Oncology (NCCN Guidelines®). The NCCN Guidelines for Patients plainly explain these expert recommendations for people with cancer and caregivers.

These NCCN Guidelines for Patients are based on the NCCN Clinical Practice Guidelines in Oncology (NCCN Guidelines®) for Uterine Neoplasms, Version 3.2025 – posted March 7, 2025.

Learn how the NCCN Guidelines for Patients are developed
NCCN.org/patient-guidelines-process

View the NCCN Guidelines for Patients free online
NCCN.org/patientguidelines

Find an NCCN Cancer Center near you
NCCN.org/cancercenters

Connect with us

Supporters

NATIONAL COMPREHENSIVE CANCER NETWORK®
NCCN FOUNDATION
Guiding Treatment. Changing Lives.

NCCN Guidelines for Patients are supported by funding from the NCCN Foundation®

NCCN Foundation gratefully acknowledges the following corporate supporters for helping to make available these NCCN Guidelines for Patients: Eisai Inc. and GSK.

NCCN independently adapts, updates, and hosts the NCCN Guidelines for Patients. Our corporate supporters do not participate in the development of the NCCN Guidelines for Patients and are not responsible for the content and recommendations contained therein.

OCRA Ovarian Cancer Research Alliance

Ovarian Cancer Research Alliance is committed to curing ovarian cancer, advocating for patients, and supporting survivors. OCRA is the largest ovarian cancer charity with over $138 million invested in research. Our international conference, webinars, and website offer the most up to date information on diagnosis, treatment and living with ovarian and gynecologic cancers. Our programs include our Patient Support line, peer mentor program, Staying Connected support series, 1:1 Counseling, scientific and psychoeducational workshops, Clinical Trial Navigator, and genetic testing program. OCRA builds community through advocacy, research, collaboration, and support. For more information, please visit ocrahope.org or call 212-268-1002.

To make a gift or learn more, visit online or email

NCCNFoundation.org/Donate

PatientGuidelines@NCCN.org

Contents

NCCN Foundation seeks to support the millions of patients and their families affected by a cancer diagnosis by funding and distributing NCCN Guidelines for Patients. NCCN Foundation is also committed to advancing cancer treatment by funding the nation's promising doctors at the center of innovation in cancer research. For more details and the full library of patient and caregiver resources, visit NCCN.org/patients.

National Comprehensive Cancer Network (NCCN) and NCCN Foundation
3025 Chemical Road, Suite 100, Plymouth Meeting, PA 19462 USA

1

About uterine cancer

The most common type of uterine cancer, endometrial, is common and can often be cured with treatment. Uterine sarcoma is a rare but treatable form of uterine cancer. Both are most often diagnosed after menopause. Surgery is recommended when possible, but other effective treatments are available if needed.

What is uterine cancer?

Uterine cancer starts when microscopic cells in the uterus change in a way that makes them grow out of control.

The uterus, also sometimes called the womb, is where a baby grows and develops during pregnancy. The cervix is the lower part of the uterus that connects it to the vagina.

The uterus has 3 main layers:

- The thin layer of tissue that lines the inside of the uterus is the **endometrium**.
- The muscular, middle layer of the uterus wall is the **myometrium**.
- The thin, outer lining of the uterus is the **serosa** or **perimetrium**.

The uterus

The uterus is where a baby grows and develops during pregnancy. It's about the size and shape of a pear, and is hollow in the middle.

The cervix is the lower part of the uterus that connects it to the vagina.

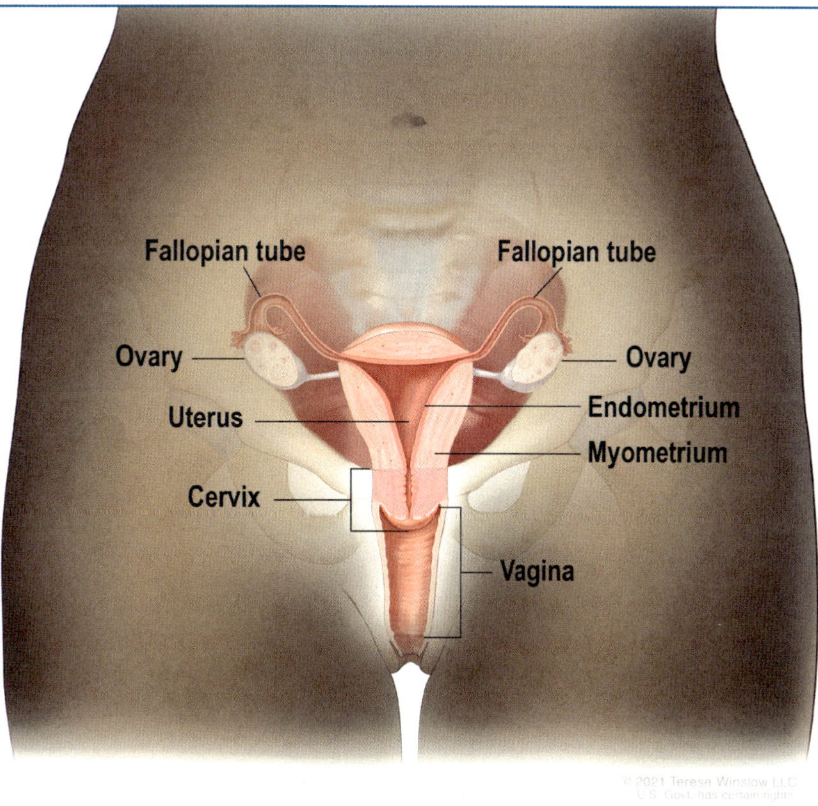

Is there more than one type?

Yes. The 2 main types of uterine cancer are described next.

Endometrial cancer

Endometrial carcinoma is common and is often found before it has spread beyond the uterus. It's called endometrial cancer because it starts in the endometrium, which is the inner lining of the uterus.

The most common symptom of endometrial cancer is abnormal vaginal bleeding. In those who are menopausal, any vaginal bleeding is abnormal and should be investigated. People who are premenopausal may have unusually long or heavy periods, but this isn't necessarily a cause for concern.

The most common type of endometrial cancer is **endometrioid**. Most of the information in this resource applies to endometrioid endometrial cancer. Treatment for less common types is also described.

A risk factor is something that increases your risk of developing a disease. Many risk factors for endometrial cancer are linked to having too much of the hormone estrogen in the body.

Types of uterine cancer

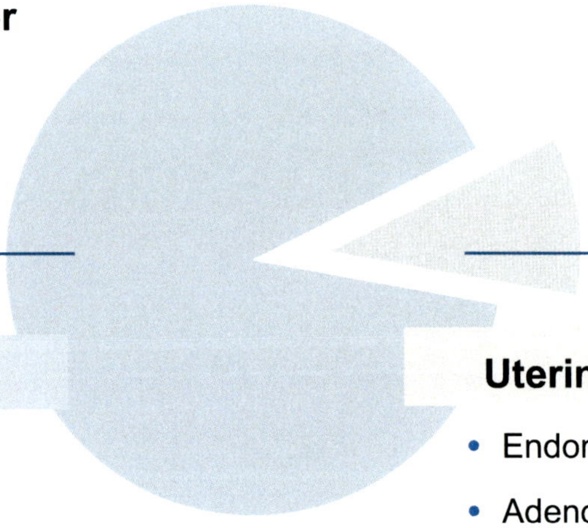

Endometrial cancer

- Endometrioid carcinoma ***(most common)***
- Serous carcinoma
- Clear cell carcinoma
- Carcinosarcoma, also known as malignant mixed Müllerian tumor (MMMT)
- Undifferentiated/ dedifferentiated carcinoma

Uterine sarcoma

- Endometrial stromal sarcoma (ESS)
- Adenosarcoma
- Uterine leiomyosarcoma (uLMS)
- Undifferentiated uterine sarcoma (UUS)
- Perivascular epithelioid cell tumor (PE-Coma)
- Inflammatory myofibroblastic tumor (IMT)

Uterine sarcoma

Uterine sarcoma starts in the connective tissue cells of the uterus. It often forms in the muscle layer of the uterus (the myometrium), or in connective tissue cells in the endometrium.

Uterine sarcomas are rare and may be harder to treat than endometrial cancer. There are different types of uterine sarcomas. See *Chapter 5: Treatment for uterine sarcoma* for more information.

How can I get the best care?

Advocate for yourself. You have an important role to play in your care. Many people feel more satisfied when they actively take part in planning their cancer care.

The NCCN Guidelines for Patients will help you play a larger role in your care. Discuss the recommendations in this guide with your care team. Ask questions about your options and share your goals and concerns.

Don't know what to ask? You're not alone. That's why we include suggested questions to ask at the end of chapters. Keep reading to find the best care for you.

How this guide can help you

Making decisions about cancer care is stressful. There's a lot to learn, and you don't know what the future holds.

Use this guide to get the information and support you need.

Patients, doctors, and other health care professionals trust the NCCN Guidelines for Patients. This guide uses clear, everyday language to explain current cancer care recommendations made by respected experts in the field. Their recommendations are based on the latest research and practices at leading cancer centers.

Your health is unique to you, so your cancer care should be, too. As you read this guide, you'll learn which treatments are likely to provide the best results for you. And you'll be better prepared to talk with your care team.

2

Testing for uterine cancer

Your care team will make a treatment plan just for you. First, they will do tests to learn about the cancer and your general health. This chapter describes the tests you may need.

First steps

If uterine cancer is suspected or confirmed, your doctor will do a complete physical exam. This often includes a pelvic exam to check the size and mobility of your uterus.

Your doctor will want to know a lot about your past and current health. They will also ask you about symptoms that could be related to uterine cancer, such as vaginal bleeding.

Biopsy

Endometrial biopsy

If you have vaginal bleeding or other possible symptoms of uterine cancer, an endometrial biopsy is typically performed. This can usually be done in your gynecologist's office.

Endometrial biopsy involves removing a sample of tissue from the lining of the uterus (the endometrium). The removed tissue is

Guide 1
Testing and care for endometrial cancer and uterine sarcoma

Necessary tests	• Ultrasound • Endometrial biopsy • Biomarker testing for POLE mutations, mismatch repair deficiency, and p53 mutations • Blood tests: Complete blood count, comprehensive metabolic panel, carcinoembryonic antigen
Other tests or care you may receive	• Cervical biopsy • Other imaging (chest X-ray, CT to look for cancer spread, pelvic MRI, PET/CT) • Genetic testing for inherited risk • Testing the tumor for hormone receptors • Help to quit smoking • Family planning and options for preserving fertility

examined by a specialized doctor called a pathologist. The pathologist determines the cancer type and subtype, when possible.

Endometrial biopsy is much better at diagnosing endometrial cancer than it is at diagnosing uterine sarcoma.

Cervical biopsy

If your doctor thinks that the cancer may have spread to the cervix, you will likely have a cervical biopsy. This is similar to an endometrial biopsy, but the cells are taken from the cervix instead of from the endometrium.

Imaging

Pelvic ultrasound

Ultrasound is good at showing the size, shape, and location of the uterus. You may have one or both of the types described next.

In a **transabdominal** ultrasound, your doctor or technician will spread a gel onto your abdomen. They will place the probe on your skin and guide it back and forth in the gel.

In a **transvaginal** ultrasound, the probe is inserted into your vagina. This may provide a better view of the uterus and nearby areas. You may feel some discomfort when the probe is inserted.

Transvaginal ultrasound

Ultrasound uses sound waves to make pictures of the inside of the body. For a transvaginal ultrasound, a probe is inserted into the vagina. Ultrasounds are generally painless, but you may feel some discomfort when the probe is inserted.

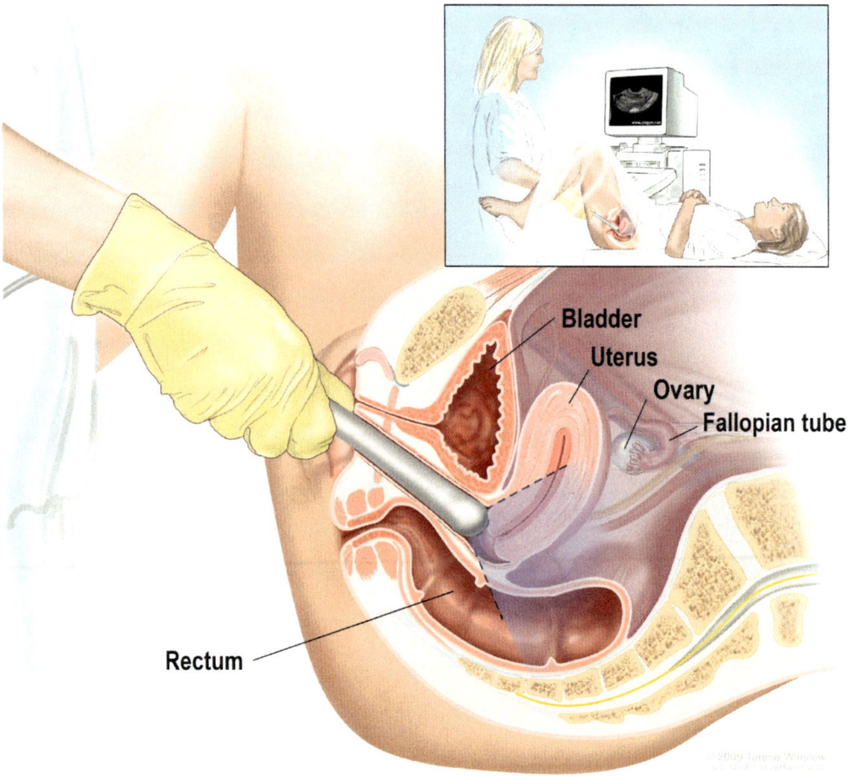

Chest x-ray

If endometrial cancer is suspected, you may have a chest x-ray. The purpose is to look for signs of disease in and around the chest. X-rays are painless and use a very small amount of radiation.

If any suspicious areas are found, your provider may order a computed tomography (CT) scan of your chest to get a better look.

CT

A CT scan is a more detailed kind of x-ray. You may have a CT scan of your chest, abdomen, and pelvis to see if cancer has spread to these areas.

During the scan, you will lie face up on a table that moves through a large tunnel-like machine. To make the images clearer, a substance called contrast may be injected into your vein. You may also be asked to drink a liquid contrast. The contrast may cause you to feel flushed or get hives.

PET/CT scan

If your doctor suspects that the cancer has spread to areas like the liver or lungs, CT may be paired with positron emission tomography (PET).

About an hour before the scan, you will be injected with a small amount of a radioactive substance, called a tracer. The tracer causes cancer cells to appear brighter than normal cells.

Distress

Depression, anxiety, fear, and distress are common after a cancer diagnosis. These feelings can make it harder to deal with cancer and its treatment. If you're feeling worried, overwhelmed, or hopeless, ask your care team for help.

More information about cancer and distress is available at NCCN.org/patientguidelines and on the NCCN Patient Guides for Cancer app.

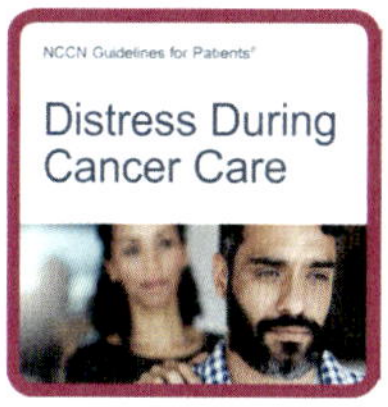

Pelvic MRI

You may have magnetic resonance imaging (MRI) of your pelvis. An MRI shows the cancer in more detail and may show whether cancer has spread to the cervix or other nearby organs. Unlike x-rays and CT, MRI doesn't use radiation.

The MRI machine is often a smaller, tunnel-like tube that can be very loud. Tell your care provider if you get nervous in tight spaces.

Testing for inherited cancer risk

Most endometrial cancers develop for unknown reasons. While rare, some people are born with a disorder that increases their risk of uterine and other cancers. Gene differences you are born with are called **germline variants.**

Families with Lynch syndrome, for example, are at high risk of developing endometrial, colorectal, and other cancers. To determine who should be tested for Lynch syndrome, the tumor is tested for mismatch repair (MMR) protein expression.

Li-Fraumeni syndrome (LFS) is a hereditary cancer syndrome that increases the risk of developing uterine sarcoma.

If an inherited cancer or cancer syndrome is suspected, your provider will refer you to a genetic counselor. This expert can speak with you and your family about testing for syndromes related to uterine cancer.

To be tested, you must provide a sample of blood or saliva. A pathologist tests the sample for inherited gene differences that cause these syndromes.

Biomarker testing

Biomarkers are features of a cancer that can be targeted for treatment. Many are mutations (changes) in your genes that are not hereditary. Non-inherited changes to DNA are called **somatic mutations**.

When possible, biomarker testing is performed on a piece of tumor tissue removed during a biopsy or surgery. If this isn't possible, a sample of your blood can be tested instead.

All **endometrial cancers** should be tested for the following biomarkers:

- POLE mutations
- Mismatch repair deficiency (dMMR)
- p53 mutations

Testing for many biomarkers at one time is called next-generation sequencing (NGS). NGS can find other rare biomarkers for which targeted treatments may be available, including *NTRK* fusions, *RET* fusions, and tumor mutational burden (TMB).

Some endometrial cancers have too much of a protein called HER2. This causes the cancer to grow and spread quickly. Testing for excess HER2 is recommended for some advanced or metastatic high-risk tumors.

All **uterine sarcomas** should be tested for *NTRK* fusions, MSI-H, *BRCA*1/2 mutations, RET fusions, *ALK* mutations, and TMB.

Hormone receptor testing

Some cancer cells have proteins on their surface that hormones can attach to. Once attached, the hormones may help the cancer grow or may help slow its growth.

Knowing whether the tumor cells have hormone receptors helps your care team plan the best treatment for you.

Testing involves analyzing a small piece of the tumor in a lab. If the tumor cells have hormone receptors, the cancer is called estrogen and/or progesterone receptor "positive."

Hormone receptor testing is recommended for most uterine sarcomas, and for recurrent or advanced endometrial cancers.

Treatment for ovarian cancer takes a team of experts. The treatment that you and your care team agree on should be noted in the treatment plan, along with possible side effects. But keep in mind that your plan may change based on new test results, new side effects, and your preferences.

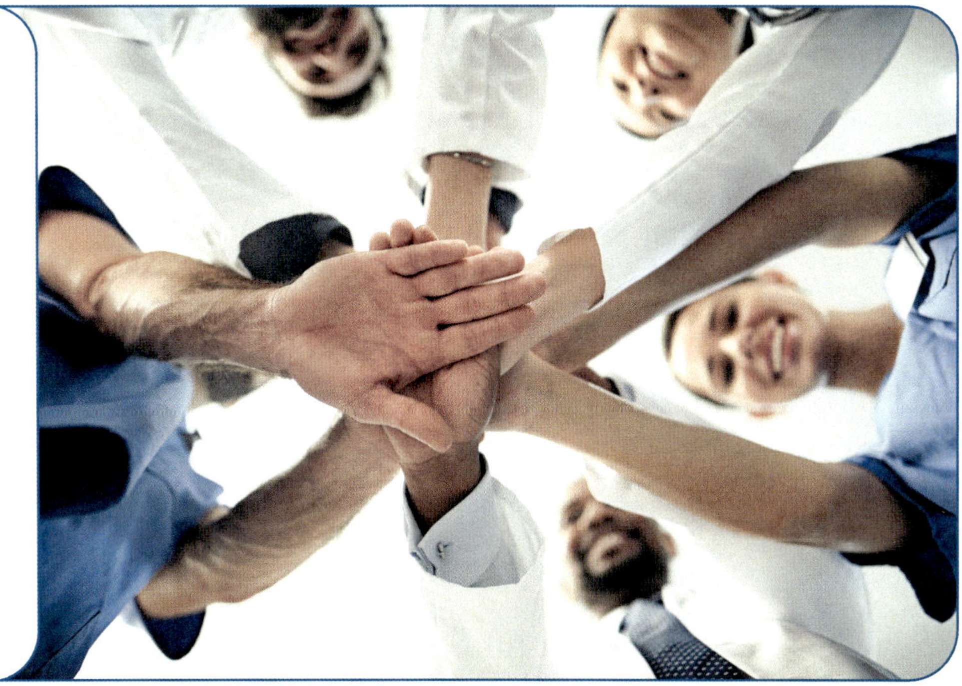

Key points

- If uterine cancer is suspected or confirmed, your care provider will do a complete physical exam and often a pelvic exam.
- Endometrial cancer is typically diagnosed by endometrial biopsy. This can usually be done in your gynecologist's office.
- An abdominal or vaginal ultrasound is often the first imaging method used to see the size, shape, and location of the uterus.
- All endometrial cancers should be tested for a biomarker (feature) called mismatch repair deficiency (dMMR).
- If the cancer has the dMMR biomarker, genetic testing for an inherited cancer syndrome called Lynch syndrome is recommended.
- Other testing before treatment includes a physical exam, health history, and blood tests. Imaging tests may also be recommended.
- Hormone receptor testing is recommended for most uterine sarcomas and for recurrent or advanced (stage 3 or 4) endometrial cancers.

Questions to ask

- I had an ultrasound. Do I need other imaging to see if the cancer has spread?
- Does the cancer have any biomarkers, such as mismatch repair deficiency or p53 mutations?
- Cancer runs in my family. Does this mean I need genetic testing?
- Does my cancer have hormone receptors? If so, is that good?

3

Types of treatment

This chapter gives an overview of the different types of treatment you may receive. To learn which of these treatments is recommended for your cancer, see the chapters that follow.

Surgery

When it can be performed safely, surgery that involves removing the uterus is the preferred treatment for uterine cancer.

Carrying a pregnancy isn't possible after a hysterectomy. If you are able to become pregnant, fertility-sparing treatment may be an option if you desire it.

Total hysterectomy and BSO

The most common procedure recommended for treating uterine cancer is total hysterectomy and bilateral salpingo-oophorectomy (BSO). Total hysterectomy removes the uterus (including the cervix). BSO removes both ovaries and both fallopian tubes.

If you are premenopausal and the cancer is only in the uterus, it may be safe for you to keep your ovaries and avoid surgical menopause. See the next page for more information on this important side effect of BSO.

Radical hysterectomy and BSO

If the cancer has grown into the cervix, you may need a radical hysterectomy. In addition to the uterus and cervix, this method also removes part of the vagina.

Total hysterectomy and BSO

The most commonly used surgery for uterine cancer removes the uterus (including the cervix), both ovaries, and both fallopian tubes.

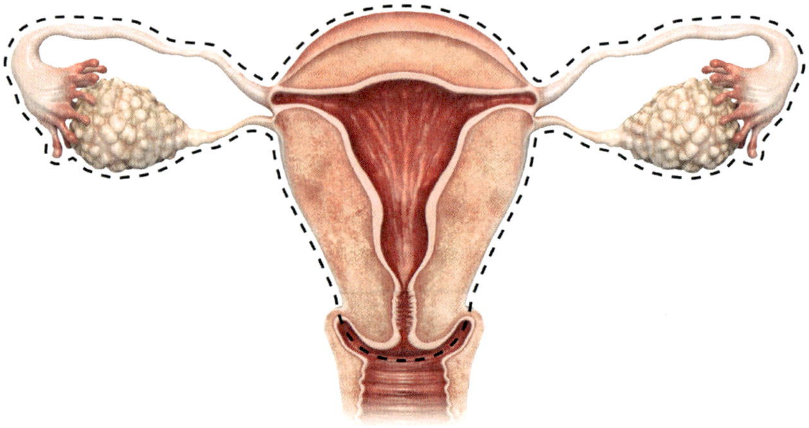

BSO to remove the ovaries and fallopian tubes is also performed. Because the cancer has spread beyond the uterus, keeping your ovaries isn't recommended. Surgical menopause, described next, will start.

Surgical menopause

Before menopause, the ovaries makes the hormones estrogen and progesterone. Removing the ovaries causes hormone levels to drop suddenly. The loss of estrogen may cause symptoms of menopause, including:

- No more periods
- Hot flashes
- Trouble sleeping
- Thinning, drying, and irritation of the lining of the vagina

Over time, the decrease in estrogen can increase your risk of heart problems and weakened bones. See *Chapter 6: Survivorship* for more information on managing symptoms of surgical menopause.

Minimally invasive surgery

Depending on the type and extent of the cancer, minimally invasive surgery may be an option This method involves making only a few small cuts into your body.

Compared to standard hysterectomy with BSO, a minimally invasive approach typically causes less pain and fewer scars. And the time it takes to recover is usually shorter.

Tumor debulking

Sometimes an endometrial tumor ends up being larger than expected, or has spread to other locations. In this case, tumor debulking may be helpful.

In this procedure, your surgeon will attempt to remove all visible areas of cancer. When safe to perform, debulking is helpful because it gives other treatments a better chance of killing leftover tumor cells.

Rely on your team

Create a personal relationship with your care team. Believe in their skills and dedication to help you. They are your greatest asset.

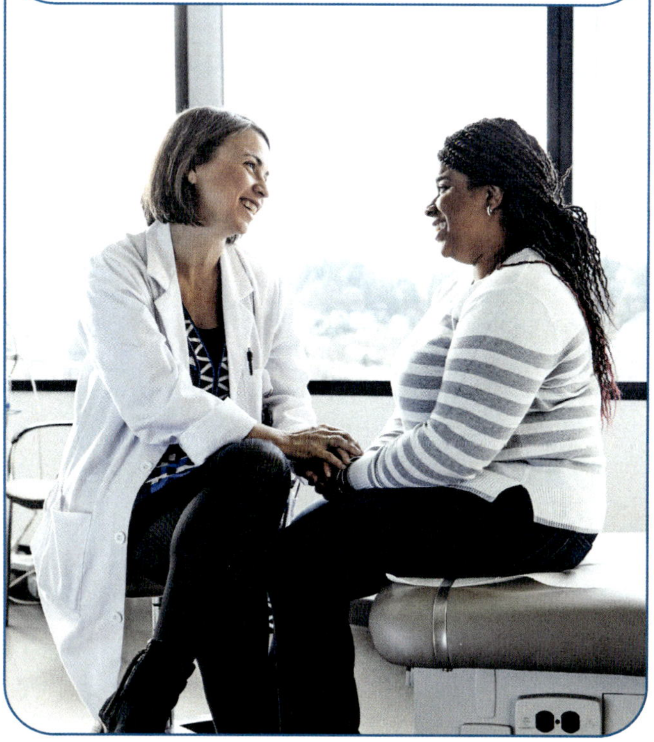

Surgical staging

During hysterectomy with BSO or other planned surgery, your surgeon will look closely at the tissues and organs closest to the pelvis for signs of cancer and take samples of any suspicious areas for testing.

Your surgeon may put fluid in the open space of your abdomen and then remove it to see if it has cancer cells. This is called peritoneal washing. They are also likely to remove lymph nodes and check them for cancer. This may be done using a procedure called a sentinel lymph node biopsy.

The information gained first-hand during surgery is used, along with tests done before surgery, to determine the stage (extent) of the cancer. This process is called surgical staging.

The main systems for staging uterine cancer consider the following features of the cancer in order to assign its stage:

- The size or extent/depth of the tumor
- Whether any lymph nodes have cancer
- Whether the cancer has spread to other parts of your body (metastasized)

Endometrial cancer stages

There are 4 main stages of endometrial cancer. Some are broken down into sub-stages that have letters and may also have a number. Examples are stage IIIB (3B) and stage IIIC2 (3C2). The stages are shown in the illustrations on the following pages.

Do I need a second opinion?

Uterine cancer is a serious diagnosis. Consider having an in-person meeting with a different doctor to see if they are in agreement with your diagnosis and treatment plan.

Stage 1 endometrial cancer

In stage 1A, the tumor is only in the lining of the uterus, or has grown less than halfway through the muscle layer.

In stage 1B, the tumor has grown more than halfway through the muscle layer.

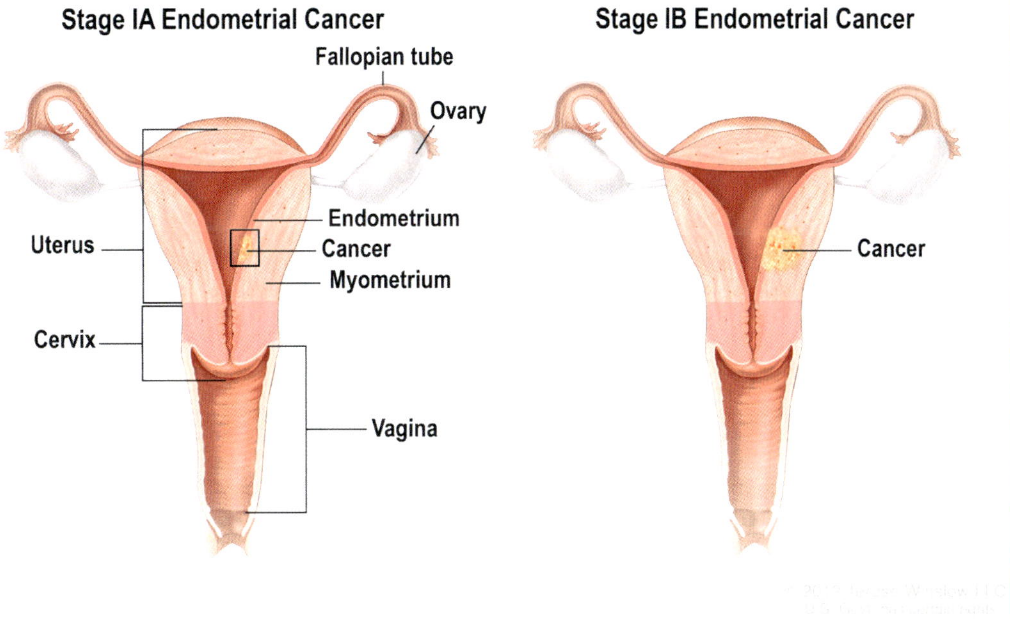

Stage 2 endometrial cancer

The tumor has grown into the cervix.

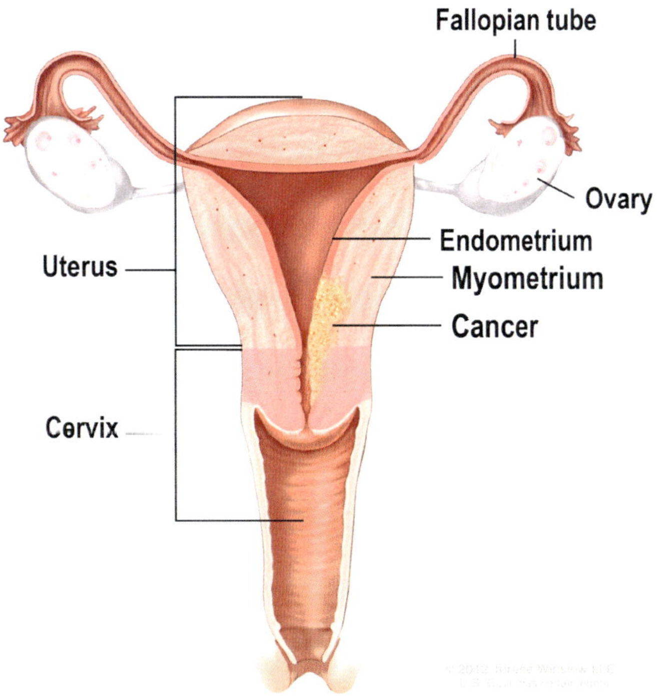

Stage 3A endometrial cancer

The tumor has grown into the outer layer of the uterus, the ovaries, or the fallopian tubes.

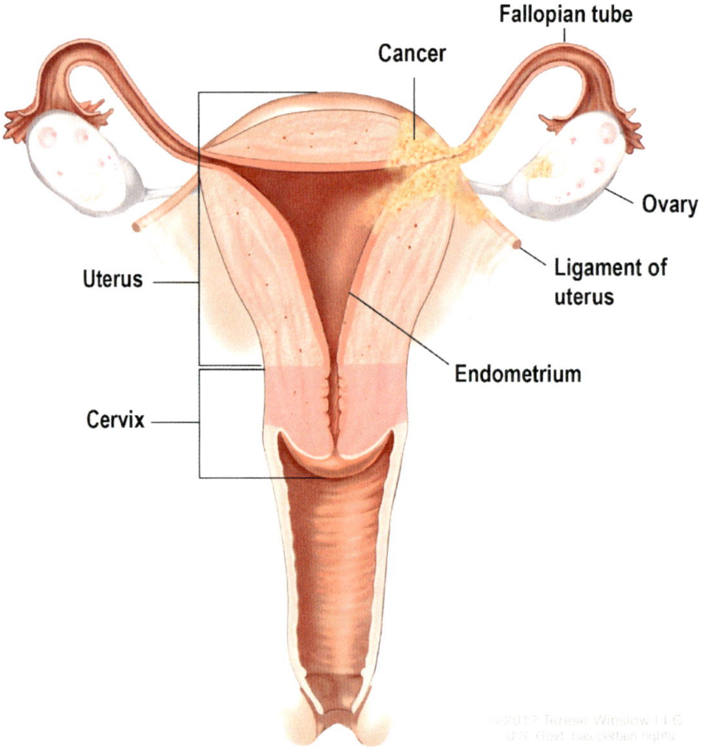

Stage 3B endometrial cancer

There is cancer in the vagina, or in the fat and connective tissue around the uterus.

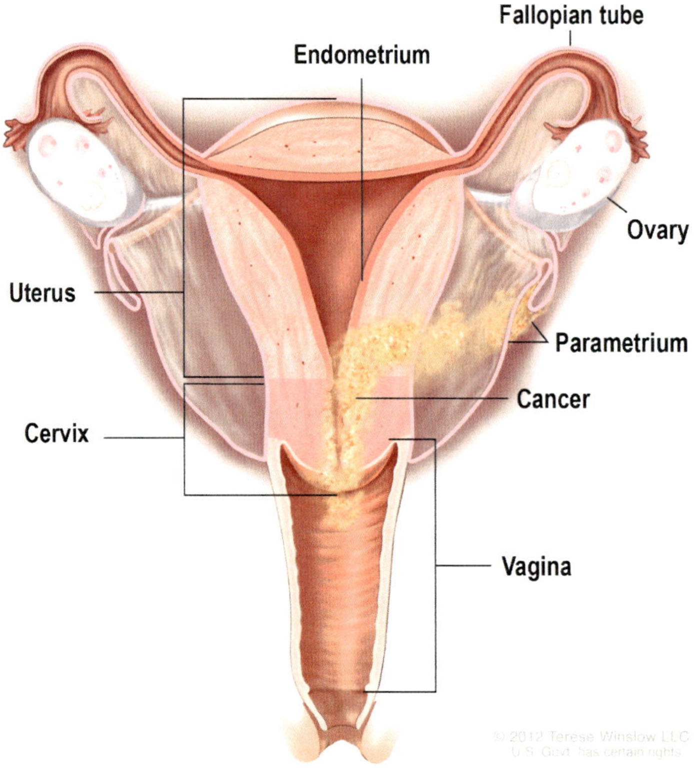

Stage 3C endometrial cancer

There is cancer in the lymph nodes closest to the uterus, called the pelvic lymph nodes (stage IIIC1) or in the lymph nodes near the bottom of the spine, called the para-aortic lymph nodes (stage IIIC2).

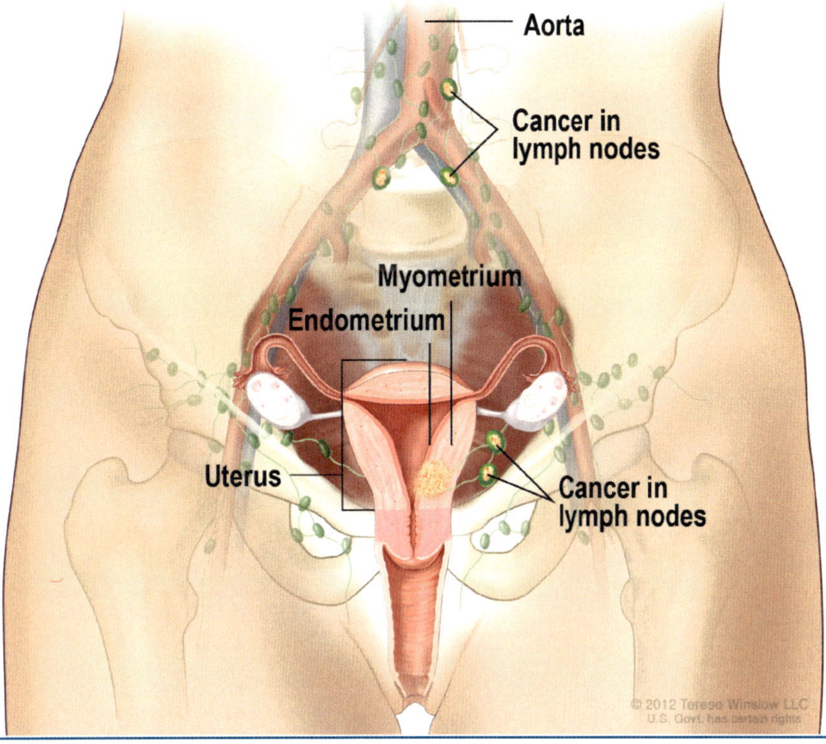

Stage 4A endometrial cancer

Cancer has spread to the lining of the bladder or intestines.

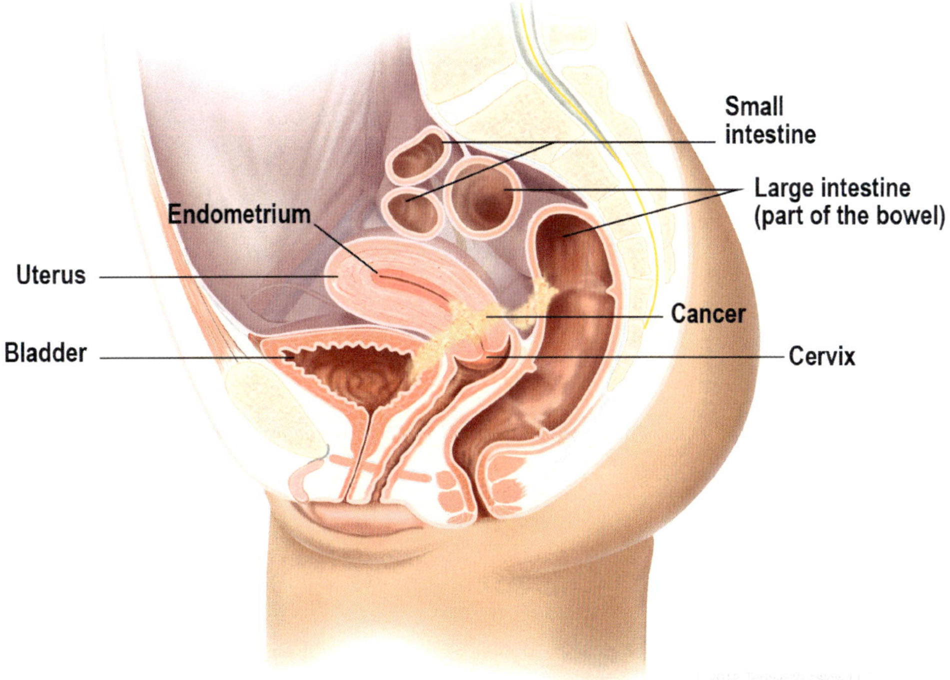

Stage 4B endometrial cancer

Cancer has spread to areas far from the uterus, such as the abdomen, the bones, or the lungs. The abdomen includes the pancreas, stomach, intestines, liver, and gallbladder.

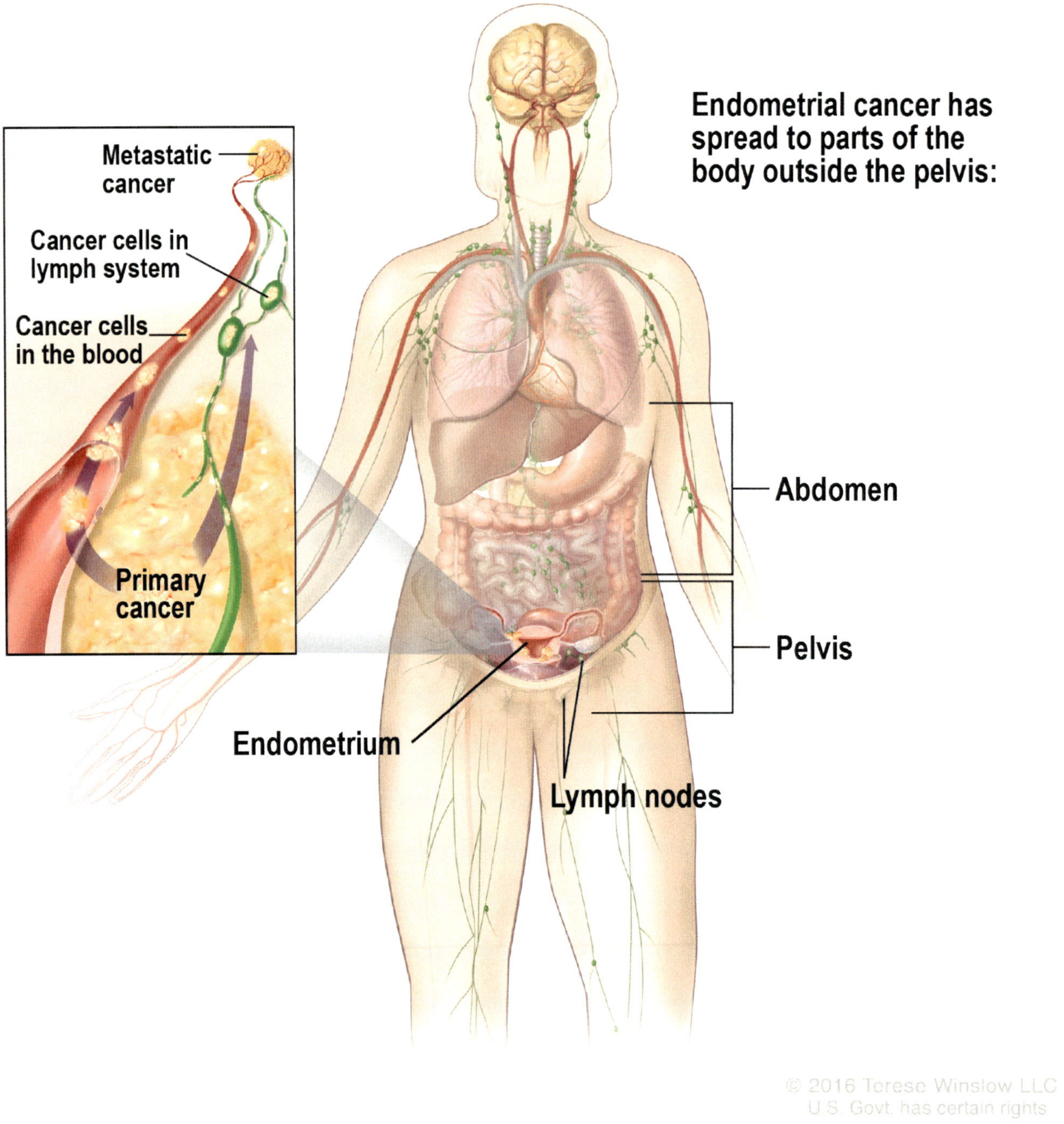

Uterine sarcoma stages

There are 4 main stages of uterine sarcoma. All of the stages are broken down into lettered sub-stages. See **Guide 2**.

Guide 2
Stages of leiomyosarcoma, endometrial stromal sarcoma, and adenosarcoma

Stage 1 - The tumor is small and only in the uterus.	
1A	**LMS and ESS:** The tumor is 5 centimeters (about 2 inches) or smaller. **For adenosarcoma:** The tumor is only in the endometrium.
1B	**LMS and ESS:** The tumor is bigger than 5 centimeters. **Adenosarcoma:** The tumor has grown less than halfway through the myometrium.
1C	**Adenosarcoma:** The tumor has grown more than halfway through the myometrium.
Stage 2 - The tumor has spread beyond the uterus, but is still in the pelvis.	
2A	The tumor has grown into the ovaries or the fallopian tubes.
2B	The tumor has also grown into other tissues in the pelvis.
Stage 3 - Cancer is in the abdomen and possibly in nearby lymph nodes.	
3A	The tumor has grown into one area of the abdomen.
3B	The tumor has grown into two areas of the abdomen.
3C	There is cancer in nearby lymph nodes.
Stage 4 - Cancer is in the bladder or rectum and possibly in areas far from the uterus.	
4A	The tumor has grown into the bladder or rectum.
4B	Cancer has spread to areas far from the uterus, such as the lungs.

Radiation therapy

There are multiple types of radiation therapy that may be recommended in addition to surgery for the treatment of endometrial cancer. The 2 most common types are external beam radiation therapy (EBRT) and brachytherapy

External beam radiation therapy

In EBRT, a large machine aims radiation (high-energy waves) at the cancer. The radiation passes through your body to reach the tumor.

To treat uterine cancer, EBRT is typically given 5 days a week for 5 to 6 weeks. One session takes about 20 minutes and the radiation beam is on for about 2 minutes. A planning session, called simulation, is needed before treatment begins. Ask your care team what to expect.

The type(s) of EBRT you may receive depends on the area of your body being treated.

Intensity-modulated radiation therapy delivers a high dose of radiation to the uterine tumor while limiting the amount that reaches surrounding normal tissue and nearby organs. This helps reduce treatment-related side effects.

Stereotactic body radiation therapy may be used to treat metastatic endometrial cancer that has spread to the liver or lungs. This method usually only requires 5 treatment sessions.

Stereotactic radiosurgery is a nonsurgical and highly precise type of radiation therapy used to treat small tumors in the brain or spine.

External beam radiation therapy

In this type of radiation therapy, a large machine aims radiation at the tumor. Some of the possible short- and long-term side effects of radiation therapy are described on the next page.

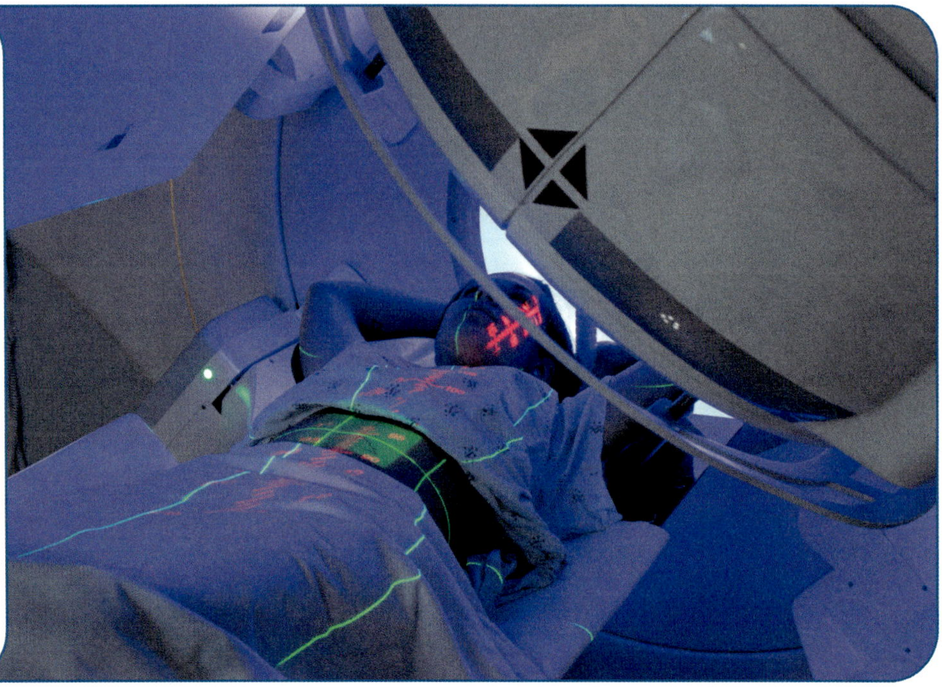

Side effects
Common side effects at the treatment site during the 5 to 6 weeks of external radiation treatment include skin irritation, tenderness, and redness.

Other short-term side effects of radiation therapy include fatigue, diarrhea, frequent urination or pain while urinating, and nausea.

Radiation therapy for uterine cancer can also have long-term and possibly serious side effects on fertility, sexual health, and bowel and bladder function. See *Chapter 6: Survivorship* for information on preventing or managing these effects.

Brachytherapy

Another type of radiation therapy used for uterine cancer is called brachytherapy. This method is also described as internal radiation therapy because the radioactive material is temporarily placed inside your body, either in the tumor itself or close to it.

Hollow tubes are placed in the vagina or uterus and a small radiation pellet travels to the region of the tumor. This may be done several times to deliver a safe dose.

Systemic therapy

Systemic therapy is treatment with substances that travel in the bloodstream, reaching and affecting all the cells in your body. Types of systemic therapy include chemotherapy, targeted therapy, immunotherapy, and endocrine therapy.

Chemotherapy is the most commonly used type of systemic therapy for uterine cancer. Most chemotherapy drugs are given by infusion. This means they are liquids slowly injected into the bloodstream through a vein.

Targeted therapy and immunotherapy are newer treatments that are most effective against cancers with specific features, called biomarkers.

These types of systemic therapy are often given in cycles of treatment days followed by days of rest. This allows your body to recover before the next cycle.

Endocrine therapy

Certain hormones (estrogen and progesterone) can affect the growth of cancer cells in the uterus.

Endocrine therapy is a type of cancer treatment that changes the levels of certain hormones in the body. It's not the same as the hormone therapy that may be used to manage symptoms of menopause, called hormone replacement therapy (HRT).

The types of endocrine therapy that may be used for uterine cancer are described next.

Progestins are lab-made versions of the hormone progesterone. They help slow the growth of endometrial cancer cells. Levonorgestrel (Mirena) is a progestin-releasing intrauterine device (IUD). Progestin pills are also available. Medroxyprogesterone acetate (Provera) is an example.

Aromatase inhibitors are oral medications that stop the fatty tissue in your body from making estrogen. This lowers the overall amount of estrogen in your body.

Tamoxifen is an oral medication used to reduce the amount of estrogen in the body. It's only used for some endometrial cancers (not uterine sarcoma).

Fulvestrant (Faslodex) blocks estrogen receptors that can cause cancer cells to grow. Fulvestrant is given by injection (shot).

Gonadotropin-releasing hormone (GnRH) agonists work by lowering estrogen levels in those with functioning ovaries.

Clinical trials

A clinical trial is a type of medical research study. After being developed and tested in a lab, potential new ways of fighting cancer need to be studied in people.

If found to be safe and effective in a clinical trial, a drug, device, or treatment approach may be approved by the U.S. Food and Drug Administration (FDA).

Everyone with cancer should carefully consider all of the treatment options available for their cancer type, including standard treatments and clinical trials. Talk to your doctor about whether a clinical trial may make sense for you.

Phases

Most cancer clinical trials focus on treatment and are done in phases.

- **Phase 1** trials study the safety and side effects of an investigational drug or treatment approach.
- **Phase 2** trials study how well the drug or approach works against a specific type of cancer.
- **Phase 3** trials test the drug or approach against a standard treatment. If the results are good, it may be approved by the FDA.
- **Phase 4** trials study the safety and benefit of an FDA-approved treatment.

Who can enroll?

It depends on the clinical trial's rules, called eligibility criteria. The rules may be about age, cancer type and stage, treatment history, or general health. They ensure that participants are alike in specific ways and that the trial is as safe as possible for the participants.

Informed consent

Clinical trials are managed by a research team. This group of experts will review the study with you in detail, including its purpose and the risks and benefits of joining. All of this information is also provided in an informed consent form. Read the form carefully and ask questions before signing it. Take time to discuss it with people you trust. Keep in mind that you can leave and seek treatment outside of the clinical trial at any time.

Will I get a placebo?

Placebos (inactive versions of real medicines) are almost never used alone in cancer clinical trials. It is common to receive either a placebo with a standard treatment, or a new drug with a standard treatment. You will be informed, verbally and in writing, if a placebo is part of a clinical trial before you enroll.

Are clinical trials free?

There is no fee to enroll in a clinical trial. The study sponsor pays for research-related costs, including the study drug. But you may need to pay for other services, like transportation or childcare, due to extra appointments. During the trial, you will continue to receive standard cancer care. This care is often covered by insurance.

Finding a clinical trial

In the United States

NCCN Cancer Centers
NCCN.org/cancercenters

The National Cancer Institute (NCI)
cancer.gov/about-cancer/treatment/clinical-trials/search

Worldwide

Ovarian Cancer Research Alliance (OCRA)
ocra.careboxhealth.com

The U.S. National Library of Medicine (NLM)
clinicaltrials.gov

Need help finding a clinical trial?

NCI's Cancer Information Service (CIS)
1.800.4.CANCER (1.800.422.6237)
cancer.gov/contact

Key points

- Total hysterectomy and bilateral salpingo-oophorectomy (BSO) is the most commonly used surgery for uterine cancer.
- The results of surgery and testing are used to stage the cancer. This is called surgical staging.
- The stage describes how much cancer there is in the body and where it has spread.
- Endometrial cancer and uterine sarcoma are staged differently. Each type has 4 main stages.
- Radiation therapy uses high-energy rays to kill cancer cells or stop new cancer cells from being made.
- External beam radiation therapy (EBRT) and vaginal brachytherapy are commonly used to treat uterine cancer.
- Chemotherapy, endocrine therapy, targeted therapy, and immunotherapy are types of systemic therapy.

Let us know what you think!

Please take a moment to complete an online survey about the NCCN Guidelines for Patients.
NCCN.org/patients/response

Questions to ask

- What are the side effects of the systemic therapy I am going to receive?
- If the cancer spreads, does the stage change?

4

Treatment for endometrial cancer

In this chapter, treatment for the most common endometrial tumor (endometrioid) is discussed first, followed by treatment for high-risk types.

Treatment for the most common type of endometrial cancer (endometrioid) is based on whether the cancer has spread beyond the uterus, and if so, how far.

When possible, surgery that includes removing the uterus is recommended. If you are able to become pregnant and want this option, you may be a candidate for fertility-sparing treatment.

Cancer is only in the uterus

If you are willing and able to have surgery, a total hysterectomy with bilateral salpingo-oophorectomy (BSO) is recommended. If you are premenopausal, it may be safe for you to keep your ovaries and avoid surgical menopause.

When possible, minimally invasive surgery is preferred for endometrioid cancer that hasn't spread beyond the body of the uterus. Ask your surgeon if a minimally invasive method is available and possible.

The results of surgery and testing are used to stage the cancer. Depending on the stage, more treatment may be needed. See page 33 for information.

Fertility-sparing treatment

Delaying surgery and treating the cancer with endocrine therapy first may be an option for a very small endometroid tumor. If progestin-based endocrine therapy kills all of the cancer, you can start trying to become pregnant.

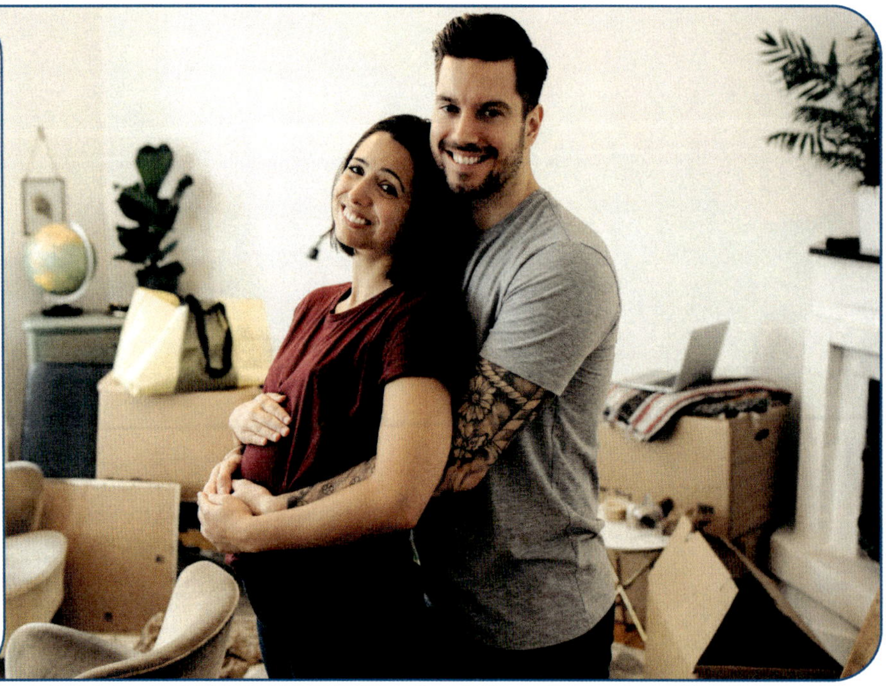

Treatment without surgery

If you can't have surgery to remove a tumor confined to the uterus, or choose not to, treatment with external beam radiation therapy (EBRT), brachytherapy, or both is recommended.

Another nonsurgical option for small endometrioid tumors is progestin-based endocrine therapy. A levonorgestrel intrauterine device (IUD), like Mirena, is preferred. Progestin pills are also a recommended option, either alone or paired with an IUD that releases levonorgestrel.

Fertility-sparing therapy

If you have a low-risk **endometrioid** tumor and want the option of carrying a pregnancy, fertility-sparing treatment may be an option. It involves delaying surgery and treating the cancer with endocrine therapy first. If this works well and kills all of the cancer, you can try to become pregnant.

Fertility-sparing therapy is only an option for **some** endometrioid tumors confined to the uterus. Ask your cancer care provider if it's an option for your cancer. If this approach is planned, consulting with a fertility expert is recommended before starting. You may also have genetic counseling and testing.

Progestin-based endocrine therapy is recommended for fertility-sparing therapy. A levonorgestrel IUD (like Mirena) is preferred. Progestin pills are also a recommended option, either alone or paired with a levonorgestrel IUD.

To learn if endocrine therapy is working, a sample of your endometrial cells will be tested

Intrauterine device (IUD)

An IUD that releases levonorgestrel is one method of endocrine therapy used in fertility-sparing therapy.

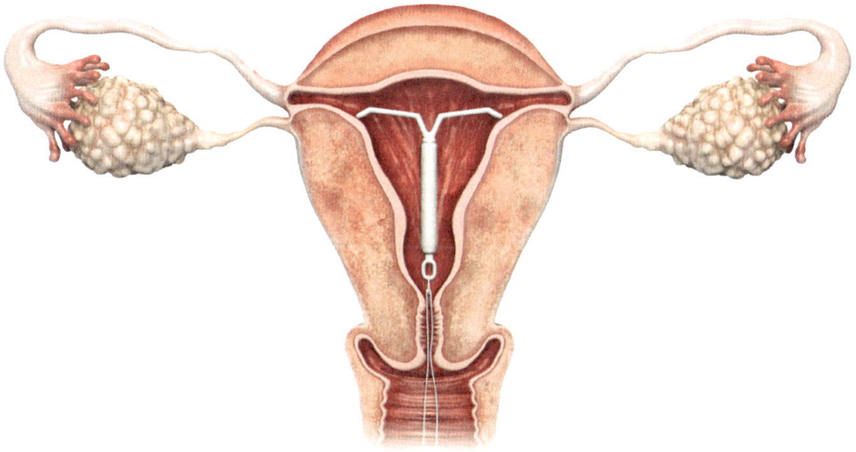

(often by endometrial biopsy) every 3 to 6 months.

If the cancer is gone after 6 months, you can stop endocrine therapy and begin trying to get pregnant. You will continue to have testing of your endometrium every 6 months.

If cancer remains in 6 months to a year, surgery is recommended. Keeping your ovaries may be an option.

It's important to maintain a healthy weight and lifestyle during fertility-sparing therapy. It may lead to better treatment outcomes. Expect your care provider to ask about the types of foods you eat, how active you are, and other habits that may affect treatment.

Cancer has spread to the cervix

If the cancer has grown into the cervix, a hysterectomy (either total or radical) with BSO is recommended. Sometimes EBRT and brachytherapy are used first to shrink the cancer before surgery.

The results of surgery and testing are used to stage the cancer. More treatment is needed for stage 2, 3, and 4 cancers. See the next page for information.

If you decline or can't have surgery first, both EBRT and brachytherapy are typically given first to try to shrink the tumor. EBRT may be paired with platinum chemotherapy. This is called chemoradiation. The chemotherapy makes it easier for the radiation to kill cancer cells.

Another option is to have chemotherapy alone first to try to shrink the cancer.

If the approach you and your team agree on works well, surgery may become possible.

Cancer has spread beyond the uterus

If the cancer has spread beyond the uterus but **not beyond the pelvis or abdomen**, total hysterectomy and BSO are recommended. Your surgeon will try to remove as much of the cancer as possible. Some people have chemotherapy before surgery to try to shrink the tumor.

The results of surgery and testing are used to stage the cancer. See the next page for information on treatment after surgery.

If the cancer has spread to areas **far from the pelvis** (metastasized), systemic therapy is recommended. At this time, the preferred regimen is carboplatin and paclitaxel. EBRT may be paired with chemotherapy.

Your cancer care provider may suggest palliative hysterectomy and BSO. The purpose isn't to cure the cancer, but rather to relieve symptoms caused by the cancer and further limit its spread. This is called palliative surgery. If surgery is planned, stereotactic body radiation therapy (SBRT) may be used to destroy small metastatic tumors.

If you decline or can't have surgery first, EBRT may be recommended for cancer that has spread within the pelvis or abdomen.

Brachytherapy, systemic therapy, or both may also be given.

If the cancer has metastasized, systemic therapy is recommended.

If the approach you and your team agree on works well, surgery may become possible.

Treatment after surgery

Recommended treatment after surgery for endometrioid cancers is described next, according to stage.

Stage 1

Your provider might recommend treatment with one or both of the following after surgery:

- Vaginal brachytherapy
- EBRT

They will consider the stage, grade, and other features of the cancer to determine if more treatment may help lower the risk of recurrence.

If you don't need more treatment, surveillance will begin.

Stage 2

Treatment with EBRT is preferred after surgery for all stage 2 endometrial cancers.

Vaginal brachytherapy is also a recommended option, and may be given alone or with EBRT.

If the cancer is very low-risk, vaginal brachytherapy alone may be considered.

In some cases, either chemotherapy or hormone therapy is given in addition to EBRT and/or vaginal brachytherapy.

Hormone therapy is typically only considered for small or slow-growing endometrioid tumors.

After any treatment(s) given after surgery, follow-up care begins.

Stages 3 and 4

The main treatment after surgery for stage 3 and 4 endometrioid cancer is systemic therapy. Either chemotherapy or hormone therapy may be used.

Hormone therapy is typically only considered for small or slow-growing endometrioid tumors.

In addition to systemic therapy, you may also have EBRT and/or vaginal brachytherapy. After systemic therapy (and radiation, if given), follow-up care begins.

High-risk endometrial cancer

Less common types of endometrial cancer can spread quickly. At the time of diagnosis, these high-risk cancers may have already spread beyond the uterus.

High-risk endometrial cancers include:

- Serous carcinoma
- Clear cell carcinoma
- Carcinosarcoma
- Undifferentiated/dedifferentiated carcinoma

Carcinosarcomas appear under the microscope as part endometrial carcinoma and part uterine sarcoma. They are also known as malignant mixed mesodermal tumors or malignant mixed Müllerian tumors (MMMTs).

Like endometrioid tumors, the first sign of high-risk endometrial tumors is vaginal bleeding. However, these kinds of endometrial cancer can also cause the following signs and symptoms:

- Lumps in the pelvis area
- Abnormal Pap smear results
- Fluid buildup or swelling in the abdomen (also known as ascites)

Testing

Testing can help determine if the cancer has spread beyond the uterus. If you haven't had imaging tests, expect to have them before treatment. Your doctor may also order a cancer antigen 125 (CA-125) blood test. A high level may mean that the cancer has spread beyond the uterus. If it has, the CA-125 level may also be checked during treatment.

For advanced or metastatic serous carcinoma or carcinosarcoma tumors, HER2 testing is also recommended.

Treatment

The most effective treatment for high-risk endometrial cancers is surgery. A total hysterectomy and BSO is recommended. When possible, minimally invasive surgery is preferred.

Fertility-sparing therapy isn't recommended for high-risk endometrial cancers. If you aren't a candidate for surgery, see page 36.

Surgical staging will be performed to learn the extent of the cancer and assign a stage. After surgery, more treatment is almost always needed for high-risk endometrial cancers. Your treatment options will depend on the tumor type and stage.

If chemotherapy is planned, the preferred regimen is carboplatin and paclitaxel. For stage 3 or 4 HER2-positive serous or carcinosarcoma tumors, a targeted therapy called trastuzumab may be given with chemotherapy.

Recommended treatment after surgery is described next, based on the tumor type.

After surgery: serous and clear cell carcinoma

If all of the cancer is removed during surgery, you don't need more treatment.

For noninvasive stage 1A disease, the results of peritoneal washing ("washings") can help guide care decisions. In this technique, the surgeon puts fluid in the open space of the abdomen and then removes it and tests it for cancer cells.

For recommended treatment after surgery according to the cancer stage, see **Guide 3**.

After surgery: carcinosarcoma

For stage 1 carcinosarcoma, both chemotherapy and vaginal brachytherapy are recommended after surgery. External radiation may also be given.

For stages 2, 3, and 4, chemotherapy is recommended after surgery. Treatment with external radiation, vaginal brachytherapy, or both may be added.

Regardless of stage, chemotherapy may be started as early as 3 to 6 weeks after surgery. Brachytherapy can be added to chemotherapy starting at 6 weeks after surgery.

Guide 3
Serous and clear cell carcinoma: treatment options after surgery

Noninvasive stage 1A	The results of peritoneal washing help your provider decide which of the following options is recommended for you: • Observation • Chemotherapy (vaginal brachytherapy may also be given) • Vaginal brachytherapy
• **Invasive stage 1A** • **Stage 1B** • **Stage 2**	**Option 1: Chemotherapy** Treatment with EBRT, brachytherapy, or both may be added. **Option 2: External radiation therapy** Treatment with brachytherapy may be added.
Stages 3 and 4	Chemotherapy is recommended. Treatment with EBRT, brachytherapy, or both may be added.

After surgery: Undifferentiated/ dedifferentiated carcinoma

Chemotherapy is recommended after surgery for carcinomas that don't fit into any specific tumor category. External radiation therapy, vaginal brachytherapy, or both may be given in addition to chemotherapy.

If surgery isn't planned first

Surgery may not be your first treatment. It may not be possible to surgically remove the cancer, you may decline to have it, or you may not be well enough to have it. In this case, there are 2 main treatment options.

One option is external radiation therapy. Vaginal brachytherapy, chemotherapy, or both may be given in addition to radiation therapy.

The second option is systemic therapy. Chemotherapy is typically given. The goal is to shrink the tumor enough to be surgically removed.

After treatment, your doctor will check the size of the tumor to see if surgery has become possible.

When treatment is over

Surveillance begins when there are no signs of cancer after treatment. It's used to find early signs that cancer has returned.

Physical exams

Physical exams are recommended on a regular basis for at least the first 5 years after treatment.

In the first 2 to 3 years, an exam is recommended every 3 to 6 months. They are needed less frequently (every 6 to 12 months) through the fifth year after treatment.

After year 5, one physical exam is recommended per year.

Other surveillance testing

If your CA-125 level was high before treatment, it may be monitored after treatment.

Other testing, including imaging, isn't recommended on a regular basis.

Other care

In addition to surveillance testing, a range of other care is important for uterine cancer survivors. This includes learning how to spot symptoms of recurrence. See *Chapter 6: Survivorship* for more information.

If recurrence is suspected

If you develop symptoms of a possible recurrence, or if your doctor notices possible signs, they will order imaging (scans). You are likely to need one or more of the following:

- Computed tomography (CT) scan of your abdomen, pelvis, and/or chest with contrast
- Positron emission tomography (PET)/CT of your whole body
- Magnetic resonance imaging (MRI) of your abdomen and pelvis

If recurrence is confirmed, see the next section for information.

Treatment for recurrence

The return of cancer is called a recurrence or a relapse. Everyone with recurrent uterine cancer is encouraged to enroll in a clinical trial for treatment, when possible.

Depending on where the cancer returns and your treatment history, your options for treatment may include radiation therapy, surgery, or chemotherapy.

Some types of endocrine therapy may be considered for treating recurrent endometrial cancer, but this is typically only recommended for small or slow-growing endometrioid tumors.

If not already performed, recurrent cancer should be tested for mutations and other biomarkers (features) that can help guide your care. See *Chapter 2: Testing for uterine cancer* for more information on biomarker testing.

Recurrence in the vagina or nearby

Endometrial cancer may return to the vagina (most common), to other areas in the pelvis, or to the abdomen.

If the new cancer growth is in an area that **hasn't been treated** with external radiation, EBRT is a recommended option. Your provider may recommend pairing EBRT with brachytherapy, systemic therapy, or both.

A second recommended option is exploratory surgery. This involves opening the abdomen to learn how far the cancer has spread and to remove all cancer that your surgeon can see. Depending on the findings, your oncologist may recommend treatment with EBRT, chemotherapy, or both after surgery.

If the new cancer growth is in an area that **has been treated** with external radiation, treatment options may include:

- Exploratory surgery
- Systemic therapy
- Lower-dose EBRT for symptom relief (palliative radiation therapy)
- Brachytherapy

Recurrence in the liver or lungs

If endometrial cancer returns after initial treatment and is found in areas such as the liver or lungs, the cancer is metastatic. It is also described as a distant recurrence. A distant recurrence isn't the same as stage 4 cancer.

If there are only a few small areas of cancer, it may be possible to remove or destroy the tumors using one or more of the following:

- Surgery
- EBRT
- Stereotactic body radiation therapy (SBRT)

If there are more than a few new areas of cancer growth, systemic therapy is recommended. The preferred chemotherapy regimen at this time is **carboplatin and paclitaxel**. A targeted therapy called trastuzumab may be added for HER2-positive serous or carcinosarcoma tumors. If you can't have paclitaxel, docetaxel is the recommended substitute.

Radiation therapy may also be given with the goal of relieving symptoms. This is known as palliative radiation therapy.

If the cancer doesn't respond or stops responding to first-line systemic therapy, there are second- and third-line options. If the tumor has any biomarkers, recommended targeted therapies are listed in **Guide 4**.

If treatment with immunotherapy is planned, see the *NCCN Guidelines for Patients: Immunotherapy Side Effects – Immune Checkpoint Inhibitors* at NCCN.org/patientguidelines and on the NCCN Patient Guides for Cancer app.

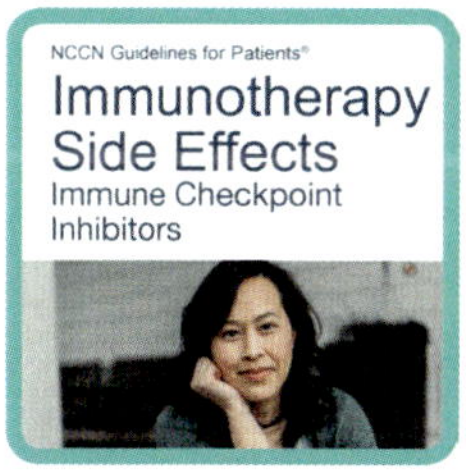

Guide 4
Targeted therapies for tumors with biomarkers

Biomarker	Available targeted therapies
pMMR (mismatch repair proficient) tumors	• Lenvatinib (Lenvima) and pembrolizumab (Keytruda) • Axitinib (Inlyta) and avelumab (Bavencio)
dMMR tumors **or** **MSI-H tumors**	• Avelumab • Dostarlimab-gxly (Jemperli) • Nivolumab (Opdivo) • Pembrolizumab • Tislelizumab-jsgr (Tevimbra) • Retifanlimab-dlwr (Zynyz)
TMB-H	• Pembrolizumab • Ipilimumab (Yervoy) and nivolumab
***RET* gene fusion**	Selpercatinib (Retevmo)
HER2-positive	Fam-trastuzumab deruxtecan-nxki (Enhertu)
***NTRK* gene fusion**	• Entrectinib (Rozlytrek) • Larotrectinib (Vitrakvi) • Repotrectinib (Augtyro)

Supportive care

Supportive care is an important part of cancer care. The goal is to improve your quality of life during and after cancer treatment. Supportive care is for everyone with cancer and their families, not just for those at the end of life. It's also known as palliative care.

Supportive care includes a wide range of services. Supportive care prevents or manages the symptoms of cancer and the side effects of cancer treatment, like pain and cancer-related fatigue. It also addresses the mental, social, emotional, and spiritual concerns faced by people with cancer.

Supportive care provides help with additional needs, such as:

- Making treatment decisions
- Coordinating your care
- Paying for care
- Planning for advance care and end of life

Read more about the types of support you may receive in *NCCN Guidelines for Patients: Palliative Care*, available at NCCN.org/patientguidelines and on the NCCN Patient Guides for Cancer app.

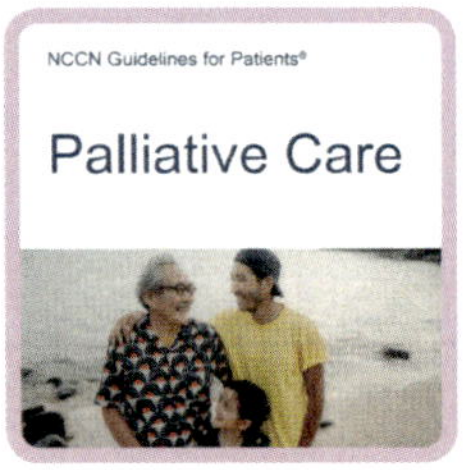

Supportive care is available for everyone with cancer. It isn't meant to treat the cancer, but rather to help with symptoms and make you more comfortable.

Key points

- Surgery is the preferred first treatment for most endometrial cancers when possible.
- If you are premenopausal and have an endometrioid tumor, fertility-sparing therapy may be an option. It involves delaying surgery and having treatment with endocrine therapy first.
- Treatment is recommended after surgery for all stage 2, 3, and 4 endometrioid tumors. Some patients with a stage 1 endometrioid tumor may benefit from treatment after surgery.
- High-risk types of endometrial cancer include serous carcinoma, clear cell carcinoma, undifferentiated/differentiated carcinoma, and carcinosarcoma.
- Follow-up care involves having regular physical exams and staying alert for symptoms of recurrence.
- Treatment for recurrent endometrial cancer depends on the location(s) of the new cancer growth and your treatment history.

Questions to ask

- I want the option of pregnancy after treatment. Am I a candidate for fertility-sparing surgery?
- I am willing and able to have surgery. Am I a candidate for a minimally invasive approach?

5

Treatment for uterine sarcoma

This chapter explains recommended testing and treatment for a rare type of uterine cancer called uterine sarcoma.

Uterine sarcoma starts in the supporting connective tissues or muscles of the uterus. Compared to endometrial cancer, uterine sarcoma tends to be hard to treat and is more likely to spread beyond the uterus.

Because uterine sarcomas are often located deep in the muscular wall of the uterus, biopsy isn't as reliable for diagnosis as it is for endometrial cancer. As a result, these cancers are often found after a hysterectomy performed for another reason.

Uterine sarcomas are sometimes found during surgery to remove fibroids. Fibroids are benign (not cancerous) tumors that grow in the uterus and cause symptoms.

This resource discusses the following types of uterine sarcoma:

- Endometrial stromal sarcoma (ESS)
- Adenosarcoma
- Uterine leiomyosarcoma (uLMS)
- Undifferentiated uterine sarcoma (UUS)
- Perivascular epithelioid cell tumor (PEComa)
- Inflammatory myofibroblastic tumor (IMT)

First steps

Imaging

Imaging tests are needed before starting treatment. A computed tomography (CT) scan of your chest, abdomen, and pelvis (with contrast) is recommended. You may also have magnetic resonance imaging (MRI) of your pelvis, abdomen, or both.

Other imaging tests that may be used to evaluate spread of cancer include combined positron emission tomography (PET)/CT scan of your neck, chest, abdomen, pelvis, and groin.

Whether you need other imaging tests will depend on your symptoms and whether your doctor thinks the cancer has spread (metastasized).

Hormone receptor testing

Until menopause, the ovaries make hormones. If the sarcoma has hormone receptors, hormones made by your ovaries may cause the cancer grow.

To help decide whether removing your ovaries would be effective against the cancer, a sample of the tumor (from a biopsy or surgery) may be tested for hormone receptors.

Hormone receptor testing is most often considered for the following types of uterine sarcoma:

- ESS
- uLMS
- Adenosarcoma

Treatment

In those with a uterus, total hysterectomy and possibly bilateral salpingo-oophorectomy (BSO) is the most effective way to treat a uterine sarcoma. If the cancer can't be removed with surgery, treatment options include radiation therapy and systemic therapy.

Sarcoma found by biopsy or fibroid removal

If the cancer is **only in the uterus**, a total hysterectomy is recommended. If you are menopausal, removing the ovaries and fallopian tubes is also recommended.

If you are able to become pregnant, you and your care provider will decide together whether to remove your ovaries and fallopian tubes (a BSO). If the cancer is hormone receptor-positive, your doctor is likely to recommend removing them.

During surgery, it is discovered that cancer has spread beyond the uterus, you may have more surgery to remove it. This decision is also made on a case-by-case basis. See Treatment after surgery on the next page.

If the cancer has (or may have) **spread beyond the uterus**, surgery will be considered. Your surgeon will consider the extent of the cancer, your symptoms, and how well the cancer can be removed with surgery. If surgery is planned, a total hysterectomy is recommended. The cancer that has spread beyond the uterus will also be removed if possible.

If you are able to become pregnant and the cancer is hormone receptor-positive, your doctor is likely to recommend removing the ovaries and fallopian tubes as well.

If you **don’t want or can't have surgery**, treatment with systemic therapy, palliative external radiation therapy, or both is recommended. Brachytherapy may be used in addition to one or both of these treatments.

Chemotherapy is often given first for systemic therapy. For tumors with certain biomarkers, targeted therapy may be an option. Recommended first-line systemic therapy options for inoperable sarcomas are listed in **Guide 5**.

Sarcoma found during prior hysterectomy

If the cancer was found after a partial or total hysterectomy, treatment will depend on the results of the original hysterectomy and whether the ovaries and fallopian tubes were removed.

If the tumor wasn’t removed in one piece or if the cervix was not removed, you may have another surgery to remove the cancer and the remaining cervix.

If you have your ovaries and fallopian tubes, they may be removed now. If only one ovary and its fallopian tube were initially removed, the remaining ovary and fallopian tube may be removed. This may be the best choice for low-grade ESS tumors, adenosarcomas, and estrogen receptor-positive tumors.

After surgery: Low-grade ESS or low-risk adenocarcinoma

If you still have your ovaries and fallopian tubes, surgery to remove them (a BSO) is recommended for stage 1 tumors. If you've already had a BSO, observation is recommended.

A BSO is also recommended for stages 2, 3, and 4 low-grade ESS tumors and low-risk adenosarcomas. In addition to surgery, one or both of the following treatments may be given:

- Anti-estrogen hormone therapy
- External radiation therapy

Aromatase inhibitors are the preferred anti-estrogen therapy for low-grade ESS and low-risk adenosarcomas. All of the recommended options for anti-estrogen therapy are listed in **Guide 5.**

If radiation therapy is used for stage 4B cancer, it is considered palliative. This means the goal isn't to treat the cancer, but to control or prevent symptoms caused by the tumor.

After surgery: High-risk adenosarcoma

If you still have your ovaries and fallopian tubes, surgery to remove them (a BSO) is recommended for stage 1 high-risk adenosarcomas. If you've already had a BSO, or if you are menopausal, observation is recommended.

A BSO is also recommended for stage 2, 3, and 4 high-risk adenosarcomas. After this surgery, your doctor may recommend treatment with chemotherapy or targeted therapy. Or, if the cancer is hormone receptor-positive, anti-estrogen therapy may be an option.

Guide 5
Anti-estrogen therapy for low-grade ESS, low-risk adenosarcoma, or hormone receptor-positive uterine sarcomas

- Aromatase inhibitors **(preferred for low-grade ESS and low-risk adenosarcoma)**
- Fulvestrant
- Megestrol acetate
- Medroxyprogesterone acetate
- GnRH analogs (for those with at least one functional ovary)

After surgery: Other tumor types

The information that follows applies to the following types of uterine sarcoma:

- High-grade ESS
- uLMS
- UUS
- Other sarcomas, such as PEComa
- Inflammatory myofibroblastic tumor (IMT)

If the cancer is stage 1, no further treatment is needed after surgery. You can start surveillance and follow-up care.

For stage 2 and 3 cancers, if the results of surgery are very good, observation may be an option. Otherwise, your provider may recommend systemic therapy, external radiation therapy, or both.

Guide 6
First-line chemotherapy and targeted therapy regimens

Preferred regimens	• Doxorubicin • Docetaxel + gemcitabine • Doxorubicin + ifosfamide • Doxorubicin + dacarbazine • Doxorubicin + trabectedin (for uLMS)
Regimens that may be used in certain cases	**For *NTRK* gene fusion-positive tumors:** • Larotrectinib (Vitrakvi) • Entrectinib (Rozlytrek) • Repotrectinib (Augtyro) **For inflammatory myofibroblastic tumors with *ALK* translocation:** • Crizotinib (Xalkori) • Ceritinib (Zykadia) • Brigatinib (Alunbrig) • Lorlatinib (Lorbrena) • Alectinib (Alecensa) **For *RET* fusion-positive tumors:** • Selpercatinib **For PEComas:** • Albumin-bound sirolimus

For stage 4A cancers, treatment with systemic therapy, external radiation therapy, or both is recommended.

For stage 4B cancer, either a chemotherapy or a targeted therapy drug is often given. Or, if the cancer is hormone receptor-positive, your doctor may recommend anti-estrogen therapy. Lower-dose external radiation therapy may be used to relieve symptoms caused by stage 4B cancer.

About systemic therapy after surgery

Most people receive chemotherapy after surgery. But if the cancer has specific biomarkers (features), targeted therapy may be a better choice.

If treatment with chemotherapy is planned, there are several preferred regimens. Most include doxorubicin (Adriamycin). Your medical oncologist will consider several factors when recommending a chemotherapy regimen. See **Guide 6**.

Surveillance

Surveillance begins when there are no signs of cancer after treatment. It is used to find early signs that cancer has returned. Physical exams and imaging tests are used to monitor for the return of uterine sarcomas. See **Guide 7**.

Guide 7
Monitoring for the return of uterine sarcoma

Physical exams	• **First 2 to 3 years:** Every 3 to 4 months • **After that:** Once or twice a year
Recommended: CT scan of chest, abdomen, and pelvis with contrast **Optional:** MRI of abdomen and pelvis and chest CT without contrast	• **First 3 years:** Every 3 to 6 months • **Years 4 and 5:** Every 6 to 12 months You may have imaging every 1 to 2 years for up to 5 more years. Your doctor will decide whether imaging should continue based on the features of your cancer (tumor type, stage, grade).

In addition to surveillance testing, a range of other care is important for cancer survivors. This includes keeping alert for cancer symptoms. See *Chapter 6: Survivorship* for more information.

During surveillance, if you develop symptoms or your provider suspects recurrence for other reasons, imaging is recommended.

Recurrence

The return of cancer after a cancer-free period is known as a recurrence. If recurrence is suspected, you will likely have imaging tests. If there is suspicion that the cancer has spread to areas far from the pelvis (metastasized), imaging may include a PET/CT scan of your neck, chest, abdomen, pelvis, and groin.

Treating a recurrence depends in part on the location of the new cancer growth. After surgery to remove the uterus, ovaries, and fallopian tubes, cancer may return to the vagina, to areas near the vagina, or to areas far from the pelvis.

Treatment of recurrent uterine sarcoma also depends on whether you've had external beam radiation therapy (EBRT). EBRT generally isn't used to treat the same area more than once.

Cancer returned to the vagina or pelvis

If **you received** prior treatment with EBRT, one of the following approaches may be used to treat cancer that returns to the vagina or pelvis:

- Surgery, with or without systemic therapy
- Systemic therapy
- Careful re-treatment of selected areas using EBRT
- Brachytherapy, with or without EBRT of selected areas

If systemic therapy is planned (alone or in addition to surgery), anti-estrogen hormone therapy is preferred for low-grade ESS and low-risk adenosarcoma.

If you **haven't received** EBRT, options include surgery and EBRT. If surgery is planned, you may have EBRT with or without systemic therapy first to try to shrink the tumor.

If treatment with EBRT is planned instead of surgery, brachytherapy, systemic therapy, or both may also be given. For low-grade ESS and low-risk adenosarcoma, anti-estrogen hormone therapy is preferred for systemic therapy.

Distant recurrence

If uterine sarcoma returns and spreads to other areas of the body, such as the liver or lungs, it is known as a distant recurrence. The cancer is metastatic. The new cancer growths, or tumors, are called metastases.

If not already performed, recurrent cancer should be tested for mutations and other biomarkers (features) that can help guide your care.

Testing for the following biomarkers is recommended:

- Microsatellite instability (MSI)
- Tumor mutational burden-high (TMB-H)
- *NTRK* gene fusion
- Inflammatory myofibroblastic tumor with *ALK* rearrangement

Minimal cancer spread

If there aren't many metastatic tumors, removing or destroying them with surgery or ablative therapies may be an option. Ablative therapies include:

- Image-guided ablation
- Stereotactic body radiation therapy (SBRT)

Ablation destroys cancer cells using heat, cold, or light-activated drugs. SBRT is a highly specialized type of external radiation requiring 5 or fewer treatment sessions.

If surgery is possible, systemic therapy, EBRT, or both may be used after surgery to kill any remaining cancer cells. If the metastases can't be surgically removed, treatment with systemic therapy, local therapies, or both is recommended. Local therapies include EBRT and ablation. If systemic therapy works well, surgery may become an option.

Many metastatic tumors

If the new cancer growth outside the pelvis is widespread, systemic therapy is recommended. Most people receive chemotherapy. There are several preferred first-line regimens.

Or, if the cancer has specific biomarkers, targeted therapy may be a better choice than chemotherapy. See **Guide 6**.

Palliative EBRT may be used in addition to systemic therapy. The goal is to shrink the tumor(s) in order to relieve or prevent symptoms.

You can also choose to have supportive care, with or without other treatment. Because the cancer can't be cured, the goal of supportive care is to make you more comfortable and to help keep the cancer under control. Supportive care may also help you live longer, improve your eating, and help you feel better overall.

Enrolling in a clinical trial may also be an option. Ask your treatment team if there is an open clinical trial that you can join. Clinical trials are discussed in more detail at the end of *Chapter 3: Types of treatment*.

Second-line and beyond systemic therapy

If the cancer does not respond or stops responding to first-line systemic therapy, other first-line regimens in **Guide 6** can be tried. Otherwise, regimens that can be tried next (second-line regimens) are listed in **Guide 8**. If the tumor has certain biomarkers, immunotherapy or targeted therapy may be an option.

Guide 8
Second-line chemotherapy and targeted therapy regimens

Preferred regimen (for leiomyosarcomas)	Trabectedin (for leiomyosarcomas)	
Recommended regimens for all other tumor types	• Gemcitabine + dacarbazine • Gemcitabine + vinorelbine • Dacarbazine • Gemcitabine • Epirubicin	• Ifosfamide • Liposomal doxorubicin • Pazopanib • Temozolomide • Regorafenib • Eribulin
Regimens that may be used in certain cases	**For TMB-H tumors:** • Pembrolizumab • Ipilimumab + nivolumab **For *BRCA*-altered leiomyosarcomas:** • Olaparib • Rucaparib • Niraparib	**For PEComas:** • Sirolimus • Everolimus • Temsirolimus **For CD4 amplification:** • Palbociclib

Key points

- Uterine sarcomas are less common tumors that start in the wall or muscles of the uterus. They are often found after a hysterectomy done for other reasons or during surgery to remove fibroids.
- Imaging tests are needed before starting treatment. A CT scan of your chest, abdomen, and pelvis with contrast is recommended. You may also have MRI of your pelvis, abdomen, or both.
- If these tests are unclear, a PET/CT scan may be ordered. Other imaging is individualized.
- For ESS, uLMS, and adenosarcomas, hormone receptor testing can help decide whether the ovaries should be removed in those of childbearing age.
- For a sarcoma found by biopsy or fibroid removal, total hysterectomy is recommended when possible. The decision to do a BSO is individualized for those of reproductive age. BSO is often recommended if the cancer is hormone receptor-positive.
- If you don't want or can't have surgery, treatment with systemic therapy, external radiation therapy, or both is recommended.

Questions to ask

- Does the cancer have hormone receptors? If so, is that good or bad?
- Who can help me manage the symptoms of surgical menopause?
- What are the most common side effects of endocrine therapy?

6

Survivorship

Survivorship focuses on the physical, emotional, and financial issues unique to cancer survivors. Survivorship begins at diagnosis and continues through treatment, recurrence, and end of life.

During and after cancer treatment, your primary care provider and your oncologist will work together to make sure you receive recommended care.

Ask your oncologist for a written survivorship care plan that includes:

- A summary of your cancer treatment history
- A description of possible short-term, late, and long-term side effects
- Recommendations on monitoring for the return of cancer
- Clear roles and responsibilities for all of your health care providers
- Recommendations on your overall health and well-being

Staying alert for recurrence or spread

Some kinds of cancer can return without giving your body any hints. If uterine cancer does come back, it often affects your body in ways that you can feel or notice (symptoms).

Your doctor will teach you about the symptoms that may mean uterine cancer has returned or spread. They include:

- Vaginal bleeding
- Blood in your urine or stool
- Loss of appetite
- Weight loss
- Pain in your stomach, midsection, hip, or back
- Cough
- Shortness of breath
- Swelling in your stomach area or legs

If you notice any of these symptoms, contact your doctor right away. Don't wait until your next scheduled visit.

Premature menopause

If you are premenopausal, surgery that removes both ovaries (or whole pelvic radiation therapy) will cause menopause. This is known as surgical menopause. It's caused by the sudden drop in estrogen in the body. This drop can cause symptoms of menopause, including:

- Hot flashes
- Sleeping problems
- Night sweats
- Weight gain
- Changes in mood
- Thinning, drying, and irritation of the vaginal lining (vaginal atrophy)

When caused by surgery, the symptoms of menopause may be sudden and more severe. There are also long-term risks of not having enough estrogen. They include heart or blood vessel problems (cardiovascular disease) and bone loss (osteoporosis).

Menopausal hormone therapy

If you have symptoms of surgical menopause and the tumor doesn't grow in response to estrogen, your doctor may suggest menopausal hormone therapy. This approach used to be called hormone replacement therapy.

If you've had a hysterectomy, an estrogen pill or patch placed on the skin is often recommended. A vaginal estrogen cream is also an option, and may be a better choice if your symptoms are mainly related to changes in the vaginal lining.

Discussion with a specialized menopausal symptom team may be helpful to determine whether this treatment is right for you.

Premature menopause

If you are premenopausal, surgically removing the ovaries or exposing them to radiation can cause symptoms of menopause, including trouble sleeping. Consulting with a menopause specialist is recommended.

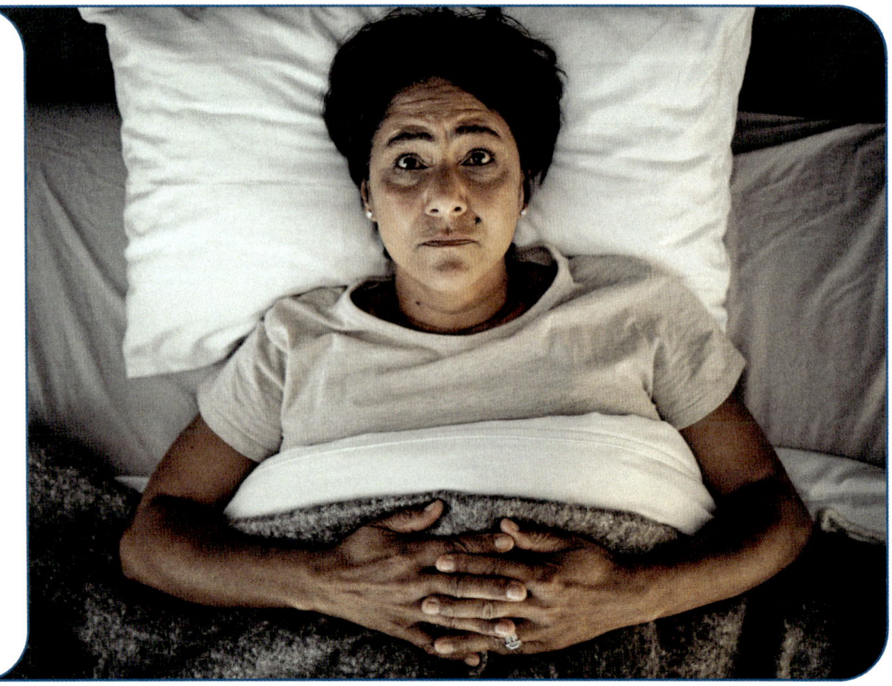

Bowel and bladder changes

After surgery or radiation therapy for uterine cancer, it may be harder to hold urine in your bladder. This is called urinary incontinence. You may also experience urgency—a sudden and strong need to urinate.

Watery and/or frequent bowel movements (diarrhea) are also possible. Pelvic floor physical therapy, described next, can help with bowel and bladder changes.

Pelvic floor physical therapy

The pelvic floor is a group of muscles that supports the organs of the pelvis. These muscles play a key role in bowel and bladder control as well as sexual function and arousal.

There are ways to strengthen these muscles before and after treatment. This is known as pelvic floor physical therapy, and there are health care professionals who specialize in it. Pelvic floor therapy can include at-home exercises to tighten and release the vaginal and anal muscles (Kegel exercises) as well as hands-on techniques by a physical therapist.

Ask your care team for help finding a pelvic floor specialist in your area.

Sexual and vaginal wellness

You may have sexual side effects after uterine cancer treatment, including:

- Reduced sex drive (libido)
- Vaginal dryness
- Pain during sex
- Narrowing and shortening of the vagina (vaginal stenosis)

Vaginal moisturizers

Older age, menopause, and some uterine cancer treatments can cause the vagina to become dry and less stretchy. To offset this side effect, use of water-based vaginal moisturizers is encouraged. Vaginal moisturizers restore moisture to the vagina and help to keep the vaginal tissue healthy. They can be used daily, and many come with applicators to make using them easier.

Vaginal dilator therapy

Radiation to the pelvic area can also cause the vagina to become shorter and narrower. This can make it uncomfortable or even painful to have sex, or to have vaginal exams by a doctor.

Using a device called a vaginal dilator during and after radiation therapy can help gradually stretch and widen the vagina. The size of the dilator can be increased over time as the vagina lengthens and widens.

Sexual health therapists

While it may be uncomfortable to talk about sexual health, keep in mind that these side effects are common and can often be managed or lessened. Consider seeing a sexual health therapist. These health care professionals specialize in helping cancer survivors and others overcome and manage sexual side effects of cancer treatment.

Many cancer treatment centers have programs focused solely on sexual health after cancer treatment. Ask your doctor about resources available through your cancer center that can help minimize the impact of cancer treatment on your sexual health.

Nerve damage

Chemotherapy can damage the sensory nerves. This is known as neuropathy. The damage can result in pain, numbness, tingling, swelling, or muscle weakness in different parts of the body. It often begins in the hands or feet and gets worse over time. Neuropathic pain is often described as a shooting or burning pain.

Lower body swelling

Treatment for uterine cancer often involves removing lymph nodes during surgery. Lymph may not drain properly after lymph nodes are removed. This can result in lymphedema. Lymphedema is swelling caused by a build-up of lymph fluid in tissues. It most often occurs in the lower body for uterine cancer survivors.

Ask your treatment team for a complete list of possible late and long-term side effects.

Mental health and wellness

The effects of uterine cancer and its treatment can be difficult to cope with. Many survivors report having an overall lower quality of life after cancer treatment. Depression, anxiety, fear of recurrence, and trouble adjusting to changes in the body are possible.

Many people also have financial stressors, such as concerns or hesitation about returning to work and insurance coverage issues. Personal relationships, sexuality, and intimacy may also be affected by a cancer diagnosis or cancer treatment.

If you are anxious, distressed, depressed, or are just having trouble coping with life after cancer, you are not alone. Tell your treatment team about these symptoms. Expect your care team to ask about your mental health. If they don't, speak up. There are resources available that can help.

Social workers at your treatment center are often excellent resources to help connect you with mental health and financial resources.

Healthy habits for cancer survivors

Follow your primary care provider's recommendations for screening for other cancers based on your age, sex, and risk level

Get other recommended health care such as blood pressure checks, hepatitis C screening, and immunizations (like the flu shot)

Eat a diet rich in plant-based foods. Limit red meat and processed foods.

Alcohol can increase the risk of some cancers. Drink little to no alcohol.

Move more, rest less. Try to exercise at a moderate intensity for at least 150 minutes per week.

Maintain a healthy weight. Tracking your weight, diet, calories, and activity levels may help you meet your goals.

Stop using tobacco. Ask your care team about options to help you quit. Counseling and medication are often options.

Radiation treatment to the pelvis increases the risk of pelvic fractures. Your provider may start checking your bone density.

More information

For more information on cancer survivorship, the following are available at NCCN.org/patientguidelines and on the app NCCN Patient Guides for Cancer:

- *Survivorship Care for Healthy Living*
- *Survivorship Care for Cancer-Related Late and Long-Term Effects*

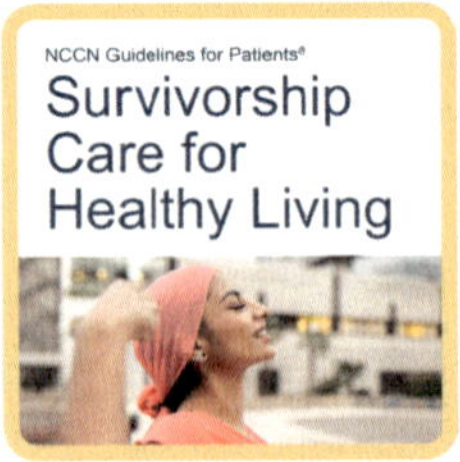

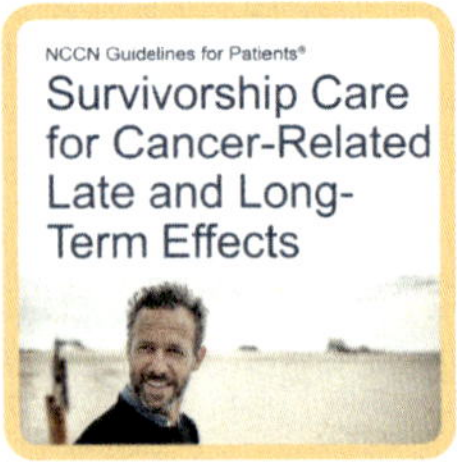

Key points

- Survivorship focuses on the physical, emotional, and financial issues unique to cancer survivors.
- A survivorship care plan is helpful in transitioning your care to your primary care doctor.
- Maintaining a few healthy habits can help prevent second cancers and other health problems.
- If you have concerns about paying for your cancer care, financial help may be available.

Questions to ask

- Can you give me a written survivorship care plan?
- Does this treatment center have a survivorship care program?
- What can I expect during a survivorship care visit?

7

Other resources

Want to learn more? Here's how you can get additional help.

What else to know

This book helps you know your options so you can make informed decisions and improve your cancer care. But it's not the only resource that you have.

Ask for as much information and help as you need. Many people are interested in learning more about:

- Managing side effects
- Genetic testing
- Building a support system
- Lifestyle changes after cancer
- Coping with other health problems

What else to do

Your health care center can help you with next steps. It often has onsite resources to help meet your needs and find answers to your questions. Health care centers can also inform you of resources in your community.

In addition to help from your providers, the resources listed in the next section provide support for many people like yourself.

Where to get help

Look through the list below and visit the provided websites to learn more about these organizations.

Bag It Cancer
Bagitcancer.org

Bone Marrow & Cancer Foundation
Bonemarrow.org

CancerCare
Cancercare.org

Cancer Hope Network
Cancerhopenetwork.org

Endometrial Cancer Action Network for African-Americans
Ecanawomen.org

FORCE: Facing Our Risk of Cancer Empowered
Facingourrisk.org

GRACE
Cancergrace.org

Imerman Angels
Imermanangels.org

Leiomyosarcoma Support and Direct Research Foundation
lmsdr.org

My Faulty Gene
Myfaultygene.org

National LeioMyoSarcoma Foundation
nlmsf.org

Ovarian Cancer Research Alliance (OCRA)
ocrahope.org

Triage Cancer
Triagecancer.org

Questions to ask

- Who can I talk to about help with housing, food, and other basic needs?
- What help is available for transportation, childcare, and home care?
- Are there other services available to me and my caregivers?

Words to know

abdomen
The belly area between the chest and pelvis.

adenocarcinoma
Cancer of cells that line organs and make fluids. Most endometrial cancers are adenocarcinomas.

ascites
Abnormal fluid buildup in the belly (abdomen) or pelvis.

bilateral salpingo-oophorectomy (BSO)
Surgery to remove both ovaries and both fallopian tubes.

biopsy
Removal of small amounts of tissue or fluid to be tested for disease.

brachytherapy
A type of radiation therapy in which radioactive material sealed in needles, seeds, wires, cylinders, or catheters is placed directly into or near a tumor. Also called internal radiation therapy.

cancer antigen 125 (CA-125)
A high level of this substance in blood may mean that endometrial cancer has spread beyond the uterus.

cancer grade
A rating of how abnormal cancer cells look when viewed under a microscope.

cancer stage
A rating of the outlook of a cancer based on its growth and spread.

carcinosarcoma
A high-risk type of endometrial cancer. Also known as malignant mixed Müllerian tumor (MMMT).

cervix
The lower part of the uterus that connects to the vagina (birth canal).

clear cell carcinoma
A high-risk type of endometrial cancer.

clinical trial
A type of research involving people that assesses investigational tests or drugs.

computed tomography (CT)
An imaging test that uses x-rays from many angles to make a picture of areas inside of the body.

contrast
A substance put into your body to make clearer pictures during imaging tests.

debulking
Surgery to remove as much cancer as possible. Also called cytoreductive surgery.

endocrine therapy
Treatment that stops the making or action of hormones in the body. Also called hormone therapy.

endometrioid cancer
The most common type of endometrial cancer.

endometrium
The layer of tissue that lines the uterus.

external beam radiation therapy (EBRT)
A cancer treatment with radiation received from a machine outside the body.

fallopian tube
A thin tube through which an egg travels from the ovary to the uterus.

genetic counselor
A health expert who has special training to help patients understand changes in genes that are related to disease.

germline variant
Gene differences you are born with.

gynecologic oncologist
A surgeon who is an expert in cancers that start in the female reproductive organs. Many gynecologic oncologists are also medical oncologists.

human epidermal growth factor receptor 2 (HER2)
A protein involved in normal cell growth. May be made in larger than normal amounts by some types of cancer cells. This may cause the cancer to grow more quickly.

infusion
A method of giving drugs slowly through a needle into a vein.

lymph
A clear fluid containing white blood cells that fight infection and disease.

lymph nodes
Small groups of special disease-fighting cells located throughout the body.

Lynch syndrome
Abnormal changes within genes that increase the chances of developing colon, rectal, endometrial, ovarian, and other cancers.

medical oncologist
A doctor who is an expert in treating cancer with drugs such as chemotherapy. Many medical oncologists specialize in specific cancers, such as gynecologic cancers or sarcomas.

menopause
The time of life when the ovaries stop producing hormones and menstrual periods stop.

metastasis
The spread of cancer cells from the first tumor to another body part.

microscopic metastases
Cancer cells that have spread from the first tumor to another body part and are too small to be seen with the naked eye.

neuropathy
A nerve problem that causes pain, tingling, and numbness in the hands and feet.

observation
A period of watching and waiting for cancer growth or recurrence.

ovary
One of a pair of organs that make eggs for reproduction and make hormones.

pathologist
A doctor who is an expert in evaluating cells and tissues to diagnose disease.

pelvic exam
A physical exam of the vagina, cervix, uterus, fallopian tubes, and ovaries.

pelvis
The body area between the hip bones.

peritoneal cavity
The space inside the belly (abdomen) that contains abdominal organs such as the intestines, stomach, and liver.

peritoneal washing
A test in which a special liquid is used to wash the inside of the belly (peritoneal cavity) to check for cancer cells.

peritoneum
The layer of tissue that lines the inside of the belly (abdomen) and pelvis and covers most organs in this space.

platinum-based chemotherapy
Treatment with two or more chemotherapy drugs and the main drug is made with platinum. Such drugs include cisplatin and carboplatin.

positron emission tomography (PET) scan
A test that uses a sugar radiotracer—a form of sugar that is put into your body and lets off a small amount of energy that is absorbed by active cells—to view the shape and function of organs and tissues inside your body.

radiation oncologist
A doctor who specializes in using radiation to treat cancer.

radiologist
A doctor who is an expert in interpreting imaging tests.

recurrence
The return of cancer after treatment. Also called relapse.

regimen
A treatment plan that specifies the drug(s), dose, schedule, and length of treatment.

reproductive system
The group of organs that work together for sexual reproduction. The female reproductive system includes the ovaries, fallopian tubes, uterus, cervix, and vagina.

serous carcinoma
A high-risk type of endometrial cancer.

somatic mutation
A non-hereditary change found in a cancer.

supportive care
Care given to improve the quality of life of people with cancer. Helps prevent or relieve symptoms caused by the cancer or cancer treatment. Also called palliative care.

surgical menopause
The stopping of menstrual periods caused by surgery to remove the ovaries.

surgical staging
The process of determining the stage (extent) of the cancer during surgery to remove the cancer.

targeted therapy
Treatment with drugs that target a specific or unique feature of cancer cells.

tumor
An abnormal mass formed by the overgrowth of cells.

undifferentiated/dedifferentiated carcinoma
A high-risk type of endometrial cancer.

unilateral salpingo-oophorectomy (USO)
Surgery that removes one ovary and the attached fallopian tube.

uterus
The organ where a fetus grows and develops during pregnancy. Also called womb.

vagina
The muscular tube through which babies are born.

washings
Sample of liquid that is tested for cancer cells after it is used to "wash" the inside of the belly (peritoneal cavity).

NCCN Contributors

This patient guide is based on the NCCN Clinical Practice Guidelines in Oncology (NCCN Guidelines®) for Uterine Neoplasms, Version 3.2025. It was adapted, reviewed, and published with help from the following people:

Dorothy A. Shead, MS
Senior Director
Patient Information Operations

Erin Vidic, MA
Senior Medical Writer, Patient Information

Lisa Diehl
Production Layout Artist

The NCCN Clinical Practice Guidelines in Oncology (NCCN Guidelines®) for Uterine Neoplasms, Version 3.2025 were developed by the following NCCN Panel Members:

Nadeem R. Abu-Rustum, MD /Chair
Memorial Sloan Kettering Cancer Center

Susana M. Campos, MD, MPH, MS / Vice Chair
Dana-Farber/Brigham and Women's Cancer Center

Sudha Amarnath, MD
Case Comprehensive Cancer Center/ University Hospitals Seidman Cancer Center and Cleveland Clinic Taussig Cancer Institute

Rebecca Arend, MD
O'Neal Comprehensive Cancer Center at UAB

Emma Barber, MD
Robert H. Lurie Comprehensive Cancer Center of Northwestern University

Kristin Bradley, MD
University of Wisconsin Carbone Cancer Center

Rebecca Brooks, MD
UC Davis Comprehensive Cancer Center

*Junzo Chino, MD
Duke Cancer Institute

Hye Sook Chon, MD
Moffitt Cancer Center

Marta Ann Crispens, MD
Vanderbilt-Ingram Cancer Center

Shari Damast, MD
Yale Cancer Center/Smilow Cancer Hospital

Christine M. Fisher, MD, MPH
University of Colorado Cancer Center

Peter Frederick, MD
Roswell Park Comprehensive Cancer Center

David K. Gaffney, MD, PhD
Huntsman Cancer Institute at the University of Utah

Stephanie Gaillard, MD, PhD
Johns Hopkins Kimmel Cancer Center

Robert Giuntoli II, MD
Abramson Cancer Center at the University of Pennsylvania

Scott Glaser, MD
City of Hope National Medical Center

Brooke E. Howitt, MD
Stanford Cancer Institute

Lisa Landrum, MD, PhD
Indiana University Melvin and Bren Simon Comprehensive Cancer Center

Jayanthi Lea, MD
UT Southwestern Simmons Comprehensive Cancer Center

*Nita Lee, MD, MPH
The UChicago Medicine Comprehensive Cancer Center

Gina Mantia-Smaldone, MD
Fox Chase Cancer Center

*Andrea Mariani, MD
Mayo Clinic Comprehensive Cancer Center

David Mutch, MD
Siteman Cancer Center at Barnes-Jewish Hospital and Washington University School of Medicine

Christa Nagel, MD
The Ohio State University Comprehensive Cancer Center - James Cancer Hospital and Solove Research Institute

Larissa Nekhlyudov, MD, MPH
Dana-Farber/Brigham and Women's Cancer Center

Karina Nieto, MD
Case Comprehensive Cancer Center/ University Hospitals Seidman Cancer Center and Cleveland Clinic Taussig Cancer Institute

*Chika Nwachukwu, MD, PhD
UC San Diego Moores Cancer Center

Mirna Podoll, MD
Vanderbilt-Ingram Cancer Center

Kerry Rodabaugh, MD
Fred & Pamela Buffett Cancer Center

Ritu Salani, MD, MBA
UCLA Jonsson Comprehensive Cancer Center

John Schorge, MD
St. Jude Children's Research Hospital/ The University of Tennessee Health Science Center

Scott Schuetze, MD, PhD
University of Michigan Rogel Cancer Center

Jean Siedel, DO, MS
University of Michigan Rogel Cancer Center

Rachel Sisodia, MD
Mass General Cancer Center

Pamela Soliman, MD, MPH
The University of Texas MD Anderson Cancer Center

Stefanie Ueda, MD
UCSF Helen Diller Family Comprehensive Cancer Center

Renata Urban, MD
Fred Hutchinson Cancer Center

*Emily Wyse
Patient Advocate

NCCN

Nicole McMillian, MS
Senior Guidelines Coordinator

Vaishnavi Sambandam, PhD
Oncology Scientist/Medical Writer

* Reviewed this patient guide. For disclosures, visit NCCN.org/disclosures.

NCCN Cancer Centers

Abramson Cancer Center
at the University of Pennsylvania
Philadelphia, Pennsylvania
800.789.7366 • *pennmedicine.org/cancer*

Case Comprehensive Cancer Center/
University Hospitals Seidman Cancer Center and
Cleveland Clinic Taussig Cancer Institute
Cleveland, Ohio
UH Seidman Cancer Center
800.641.2422 • *uhhospitals.org/services/cancer-services*
CC Taussig Cancer Institute
866.223.8100 • *my.clevelandclinic.org/departments/cancer*
Case CCC
216.844.8797 • *case.edu/cancer*

City of Hope National Medical Center
Duarte, California
800.826.4673 • *cityofhope.org*

Dana-Farber/Brigham and Women's Cancer Center |
Mass General Cancer Center
Boston, Massachusetts
877.442.3324 • *youhaveus.org*
617.726.5130 • *massgeneral.org/cancer-center*

Duke Cancer Institute
Durham, North Carolina
888.275.3853 • *dukecancerinstitute.org*

Fox Chase Cancer Center
Philadelphia, Pennsylvania
888.369.2427 • *foxchase.org*

Fred & Pamela Buffett Cancer Center
Omaha, Nebraska
402.559.5600 • *unmc.edu/cancercenter*

Fred Hutchinson Cancer Center
Seattle, Washington
206.667.5000 • *fredhutch.org*

Huntsman Cancer Institute at the University of Utah
Salt Lake City, Utah
800.824.2073 • *healthcare.utah.edu/huntsmancancerinstitute*

Indiana University Melvin and Bren Simon
Comprehensive Cancer Center
Indianapolis, Indiana
888.600.4822 • *www.cancer.iu.edu*

Johns Hopkins Kimmel Cancer Center
Baltimore, Maryland
410.955.8964
www.hopkinskimmelcancercenter.org

Mayo Clinic Comprehensive Cancer Center
Phoenix/Scottsdale, Arizona
Jacksonville, Florida
Rochester, Minnesota
480.301.8000 • *Arizona*
904.953.0853 • *Florida*
507.538.3270 • *Minnesota*
mayoclinic.org/cancercenter

Memorial Sloan Kettering Cancer Center
New York, New York
800.525.2225 • *mskcc.org*

Moffitt Cancer Center
Tampa, Florida
888.663.3488 • *moffitt.org*

O'Neal Comprehensive Cancer Center at UAB
Birmingham, Alabama
800.822.0933 • *uab.edu/onealcancercenter*

Robert H. Lurie Comprehensive Cancer Center
of Northwestern University
Chicago, Illinois
866.587.4322 • *cancer.northwestern.edu*

Roswell Park Comprehensive Cancer Center
Buffalo, New York
877.275.7724 • *roswellpark.org*

Siteman Cancer Center at Barnes-Jewish Hospital
and Washington University School of Medicine
St. Louis, Missouri
800.600.3606 • *siteman.wustl.edu*

St. Jude Children's Research Hospital/
The University of Tennessee Health Science Center
Memphis, Tennessee
866.278.5833 • *stjude.org*
901.448.5500 • *uthsc.edu*

Stanford Cancer Institute
Stanford, California
877.668.7535 • *cancer.stanford.edu*

The Ohio State University Comprehensive Cancer Center -
James Cancer Hospital and Solove Research Institute
Columbus, Ohio
800.293.5066 • *cancer.osu.edu*

The UChicago Medicine Comprehensive Cancer Center
Chicago, Illinois
773.702.1000 • *uchicagomedicine.org/cancer*

The University of Texas MD Anderson Cancer Center
Houston, Texas
844.269.5922 • *mdanderson.org*

UC Davis Comprehensive Cancer Center
Sacramento, California
916.734.5959 • 800.770.9261
health.ucdavis.edu/cancer

UC San Diego Moores Cancer Center
La Jolla, California
858.822.6100 • cancer.ucsd.edu

UCLA Jonsson Comprehensive Cancer Center
Los Angeles, California
310.825.5268 • uclahealth.org/cancer

UCSF Helen Diller Family
Comprehensive Cancer Center
San Francisco, California
800.689.8273 • cancer.ucsf.edu

University of Colorado Cancer Center
Aurora, Colorado
720.848.0300 • coloradocancercenter.org

University of Michigan Rogel Cancer Center
Ann Arbor, Michigan
800.865.1125 • rogelcancercenter.org

University of Wisconsin Carbone Cancer Center
Madison, Wisconsin
608.265.1700 • uwhealth.org/cancer

UT Southwestern Simmons
Comprehensive Cancer Center
Dallas, Texas
214.648.3111 • utsouthwestern.edu/simmons

Vanderbilt-Ingram Cancer Center
Nashville, Tennessee
877.936.8422 • vicc.org

Yale Cancer Center/Smilow Cancer Hospital
New Haven, Connecticut
855.4.SMILOW • yalecancercenter.org

share with us.

Take our survey and help make the NCCN Guidelines for Patients better for everyone!

NCCN.org/patients/comments

Notes

Index

Made in the USA
Coppell, TX
23 December 2025

67239385R00043